INNER ALCHEMY

A No-Holds-Barred Guide to Understanding

Your Body and Reclaiming Your Health

Dr. Nicholas James Nelson

Copyright © 2024 Dr. Nicholas James Nelson.

For my Parents
For my Mom, for being my reason why.
For my Dad, for being my example.

Table of Contents

FOREWORD FROM THE AUTHOR

I have no idea if this book will make it into many hands outside of my own or if it won't. If it does, awesome, and if it doesn't, that's ok too. Writing this was a life goal of mine, and that's what's most important. I remember the exact time and place where I decided that I wanted to become a writer. If that transpires into a career in writing, that's even better, but what is most important to me is that I did what I said I would do and what I dreamed I would do.

This book is incredibly important to me. Not just because it is the fulfillment of one of my biggest dreams but because the information inside of it represents over a decade of passion, experience, and insights into the biggest questions I have always had: Who are we, what are we doing here, and what is the experience of life itself? These questions have guided my career, time, and pursuits throughout this life, and I continue to do so daily. This is not a complete or exhaustive encyclopedia of information I have acquired, nor is it unchanging. This is a summary of what I could put together over a few of the most stressful years in our lifetimes and through the skills of a first-time writer. What is written within are the intellectual musings of a free-thinking individual. The ideas and opinions I pose are not written as a clinically licensed chiropractor; nor are they intended to be taken as medical advice. Instead, they are opinions and ideas of a free-thinking member of society who is searching for the answers to the questions stated above, and how they apply to our own health.

Though the information in this book sometimes may not flow seamlessly, I believe everything mentioned within is important and insightful enough to be included. My only hope is that the reader, whoever and however many there may be, forgives me for the holes I have left and understands that this is only the beginning of this project of passion and that I still have much to learn about the art of writing, and even more left to discover of the stubborn mysteries within the human body. I also hope that as time goes on, I can continue to work toward these ideals and share what I find along the way. Thank you for joining me on this journey.

Please, enjoy.

Dr. Nicholas James Nelson

INTRODUCTION

The recent years have been filled with an absolute whirlwind of information. Some have called it the great awakening, while others refer to it as the time of unveiling. I think both are accurate but also, in some ways, inadequate. I began writing this book before the world flipped on its head and the chaos of corruption erupted to its current deafening volume. Though this has made the information in this text all the more valuable, it has made writing and completing it no quick and simple task.

From the time I began composing material for this text in 2018 to the final publication date in 2024, the world as we knew it had changed in so many ways that it was almost unimaginable. To stay as relevant and current as possible, the content of this book had to be constantly modified and updated along the way to maintain its relevance and accuracy in its final form. In some ways, these changes have proven to be helpful as I believe the world is more ready than ever to accept the information written on these pages, but in others, I am still uncertain how many readers will be open enough to accept the information within as truth. Though the base content of the book did not change much from its original form, the events of the world helped bring to light just how and why this information is so desperately needed now more than ever.

For this divine timing, I feel blessed and hopeful that the insights held within may have the capacity to help each of us claw our way out of the darkest age of health and science we have seen in modern recorded history and back into a place of empowerment and self-understanding.

Living through our recent global pandemic has been incredibly challenging; however, it seems it has also unintentionally catalyzed a global awakening. Things that were only suspected behind closed doors by small groups of societal outcasts have been exposed to the world in their true, naked forms. These exposures, and all the subsequent coordinated responses that followed them, have provided a platform in which we have been able to witness so many areas of our society and culture slowly become see-through. The holes in the fabric of the human story have begun to show. For those that have the eyes to see, we are witnessing its very foundations being ripped open at an alarming speed, revealing many ugly and uncomfortable truths along the way.

The veil is lifting.

Daily. Weekly. Yearly. As time seems to be speeding by on fast forward, we are slowly discovering that everything we thought we knew about our lives and the world we live in has been nothing more than a carefully crafted story held up by a shit ton of money, lies, and power.

We are realizing that the culture, social fabric, and history that we were all taught to believe may not be quite as true as we were avidly told. Political parties and their corruption have become so glaringly obvious that it's hard for many people to comfortably vote in one direction or the other. Companies and campaigns that, on the surface, have been set up to help specific groups or causes are showing themselves to be insidious organizations perfectly situated to covertly perform vomit-inducing tasks, safely masked in the façade of their charity. Our so-called freedom is shrinking by the day, and the reasons for each new mandate, tax, or restriction have no actual basis in scientific evidence or vetted procedures; rather, they are shotgun political decisions that the public and unbiased professionals seem to have no say in whatsoever, regardless of the alleged democracy we are told we are living in.

Though some of these pandemic restrictions have eased since the beginning of writing this book, the unrelenting movement in the background to form a One World Government is still very much on schedule and progressing rapidly.

As we watch these areas of our society break down, there is something that is slowly becoming clear: Science, especially when combined with political power, money, and the potential for control, is not the pure and unbiased pursuit of truth and progression of intellect it has been touted to be. It is not the white knight that has been sent to deliver us from dogma and superstition and lead us in the direction of unfiltered human and technological innovation. Instead, science has *become* the dogma, bringing its own imposed superstitions with it. Science, especially medical science in its current use, is just a tool used to elevate those who have purchased its endorsement and benefit from its conclusions and destroy and defame those who cannot or will not play the same game.

Simply stated, science has become a tool for manipulation and control, and it is *bought and paid for*. This fact is hard for many to accept, just like it is hard to turn against the faith in which you were raised. The irony, however, is that science actually *is* the faith in which our generation was raised. We live in a time when religion has become a dirty word, and science has been elevated to fill the authoritarian role that religion once had. It has become our unquestioned hope and savior, along with the same commands that if we even consider questioning it, we will suffer eternal consequences. We have thousands of confused people touting the war cries of the scientific era, like "Show me your sources," "Is that from a peer-reviewed journal," "There is no science to prove that," or the most trendy and currently degrading choice: "That's just a conspiracy," all the while puffing out their chests with a sense of superior intellect even though they have never spent a single minute of their time in the pursuits of an honest, curious, and unbiased stint of research, choosing instead to obediently regurgitate the rhetoric that has been fed to them by the coordinated efforts of the media and designated authorities.

Gross.

This needs to change, and we need to be the ones that change it.

If we are going to successfully unravel the web of lies we are hopelessly stuck in, we need a new lens to look through. As Albert Einstein once said: "You can't fix a problem using the same level of thinking that created it." So, to solve this seemingly hopeless mess, we need to change our thinking. We need to change our understanding of who and what we are and what it really means to be a healthy human.

HOW I GOT HERE

I have studied the human body for over 16 years across multiple specialty fields. It all began with an obsession with fitness and human performance, which led me to work as a personal trainer for five years before moving on to formal university and higher education. My position as a personal trainer, combined with an obsessive mind, provided me with a solid platform to begin my scientific and academic pursuits through avidly searching for the latest and greatest way to train, eat, supplement for performance enhancement and to bio-hack my system into high-quality muscle and power development. I read as much literature as possible from leading health experts and fitness gurus, looking for any information that could make me healthier, stronger, more aesthetic, and better at my job. This was my first glance into the alarming world of health science.

After a few years of this, I came to the disturbing realization that the majority of fitness programs, health advice, and nutritional advice handed out in fitness magazines, blogs, websites, books, and digital media alike, even when being provided by experts around me to their unknowing and trusting clients, were absolute loads of bullshit.

Extremely unhealthy tips and tricks are being pushed by fitness professionals who are being paid to push them but have actually never used them a day in their lives. A perfect example of this can be seen in common home gym commercials that feature an unbelievably muscular individual who has clearly spent hours upon hours, week after week, for *years* training and sculpting their physique, only to come on the screen and sell the home gym by alluding that it is the sole reason and piece of equipment used to help them look the way they do.

Another example comes from advice from a famous fitness and cover model I will leave unnamed. Before I go on, I would like to say that this individual was an incredible inspiration to many, including myself. He had one of the most balanced and aesthetic physiques of anyone in the industry and spoke a lot about the psychological and mental sides of training and life. He was one of the most significant and influential fitness models of my time and one that, on many occasions, motivated me to get my ass to the gym on tough days. Now, with all that said, one thing he claimed he did and, still to this day, I can't wrap my head around, was not actually eating any solid food, and instead promoted the idea of drinking an exclusively liquid diet of his specific sponsored brand of protein shake. Convenient.

Now, hear me out. I know that you can, in theory, put a ton of nutrients into a protein shake and make some clean and healthy meal replacements, but telling the average – or elite individual, for that matter, to live off of shakes alone goes against every fiber of my being, and all of human evolution. It's like the adult version of the formula vs. breast milk debate. With all other factors eliminated, when looking at the two options for overall health and bioavailability of nutrients, there is really no comparison. Whether he actually lived this way and for how long, I will never know, but it was what he claimed on more than one occasion, with the reason being cited that it eliminates the stress of digesting solid food on the body. This proves that an individual can be highly qualified and highly successful in a certain area of expertise and still push a bad idea.

These are just two examples that are present in our current health and fitness industry that influence and guide the public but are also obviously selling a product. You may be thinking, "This is what marketing is about; there is nothing wrong with that," and you may be right. But what about the official, government, and medically sanctioned recommendations on our diet? I mean, if a badass and chiseled Greek God isn't giving us real and healthy recommendations, then we should be able to at least fall back on the food guidelines pushed by our governments that our entire public health and food recommendations are built on, right?

Right?

Wrong.

Sadly, very wrong.

FOOD PYRAMID – PAY TO PLAY

The American and Canadian standard food guides (you know, the ones you were taught in elementary school that look like a pyramid made up of different layers of food groups based on importance in our diet) were sadly never created based on any research, any common knowledge or any formal history of health and food consumption across any parts of the world. As much as we would all like to hope that there was actual scientific research involved in these food guides, it turns out there wasn't.

Instead, do you want to know how the United States Department of Agriculture made the magic food guide that has been used to develop our basic rules of nutrition for roughly the last 30 years?

Lobbying.

Competitive lobbying by the various food industries, mainly from the dairy and cereal industries as the top bidders, is *what determined North America's dietary guidelines for over three decades.*

Yes, you heard that right. Our food guide provides our recommendations as to how much of each type of food to consume daily based *in proportion* to how much those specific industries were willing to pay the United States Department of Agriculture (USDA). This was a bought and paid-for advertising campaign that was spread across all North America, and from 1992 until January of 2019 in Canada and 2020 in the United States, and was used as the basis of dietary recommendations by the official doctors and experts. In fact, a poster of this food pyramid can be found at almost every local GP doctor's office still to this day, along with the BMI body composition chart that labels me, an individual who is currently 5"10 and 190lbs, as borderline obese.[1]

Now, just take a second and really think about that. Think about the implications of this and how many good-intentioned parents and

---

[1] An extensive look at the history of the food pyramid can be found in the book called "Death by Food Pyramid: How Shoddy Science, Sketchy Politics, and Shady Special Interests Have Ruined Our Health" by Denise Minger.

unknowing children used this guide to diligently feed their families and themselves in an attempt to be as healthy as possible, based not on what would lead to better health but instead on which industry paid more.

Now, just when you think it can't get worse than that, in 2022, the U.S. released an updated food guide, which lists Fruit Loops, the sugary, colorful cereal of Toucan Sam, as a healthier option than grass-fed beef, eggs, meat, and dairy… No, I'm not joking.

Fruit Loops is now considered healthier than all the foods humans have survived on for the entire history of our species. Do we see a problem?

WE HAVE BEEN LED ASTRAY

I should get a few things off my chest and into the open before continuing. First, I'm tired of the abundance of people who consider themselves experts in their field and go on to write and talk as public influencers yet have only the faintest idea of what is going on in their so-called area of expertise. Second, I am tired of the mass amount of false, incomplete, or straight-up fabricated information being spread by government agencies, social media, mainstream media, and supposed experts alike. This pandemic of bullshit has resulted in a state of confusion in our culture, unlike anything we have ever witnessed before.

We live in an information age, and despite the benefit of this when used consciously, it has its downsides. Specifically, it means that every person who has internet access is constantly and unrelentingly bombarded with information that is designed to grab your specific interest and lead you away from anything that can provide you a sense of true meaning or true health. Nothing in this world is about the betterment of the people anymore. The capitalist dream has run rampant, morphing into a pseudo-communism where you are hard-pressed to find any true information that can help you become empowered, independent, and self-sufficient. At least not anywhere in the mainstream.

Think about it: As a society run by corporate lobbying and multibillion-dollar companies, the only way to maintain the status quo is for you, the everyday Jane or Joe, to remain oblivious, distracted, scared, and buying their shit.

Reaction and distraction.

Capitalism was supposed to facilitate the land of opportunity, and monopolies were supposed to be illegal. The only problem with this is monopolies make money, and capitalism is about making money.

Every person for themselves.

Here's the catch, though: these patterns do not just remain contained in board rooms and tall towers.

People with power want more power. People with money want more money. Once you are at the front of the line where everyone behind you would take your place in a heartbeat, you begin to set up safeguards to ensure that can never happen. You begin to play the defensive game. You begin to build into the system fundamental insurances that guarantee you will never lose your place, and the people behind you are moved to a different line entirely.

Of course, every reasonable person understands this logic to some degree; however, the part that interests me is that everyone seems to believe there is some definite line these tendencies do not cross because of a perceived universal ethics. It's an almost chosen ignorance to believe that corruption can work in all areas of the underbelly of life, but anything to do with health and human sovereignty would definitely be safeguarded by an imaginary forcefield that keeps all this scummy behavior outside, despite these industries being multi-trillion-dollar industries with higher earning potentials than even oil and gold.

There is the belief that all doctors are doctors because they have an overwhelming sense of right and wrong and believe it is their moral obligation to help people. The paycheck attached to that doesn't matter to them. We also believe that the massive companies that write their paychecks and design the drugs prescribed by these ethical superheroes are an organization of Gandhi-like geniuses working tirelessly to solve world illness and suffering. Oh, and of course, the governing bodies that license and support these doctors are run by straight-shooting righteous individuals who are here to be the rightful gatekeepers of health for the human race, guided only by pristine levels of morals and social values.

We are made to believe that these companies that have access to billions of dollars want to spend it all graciously on curing the ailments of us lowly citizens whose illnesses have served as the very funding for their aforementioned billions.

This blind spot in good people like you or me has allowed organizations like cancer research foundations the ability to set up smoke screen advertisements to guilt you into donating to them while they happily pocket the profit, knowing full well that any cancer treatment that is discovered that cannot be patented and provide a return on investment larger than the funding they are getting through donations will never be allowed to see the light of day… and it hasn't.

Think about it logically for a second as a business owner. Suppose the cancer research industry is a multi-billion-dollar industry, with hundreds of thousands of people employed to run, oversee, and manage the research, charities, and marketing campaigns for donations. What happens to those people when the cure – as if there is a single cure – is found? Especially if it is a really good one?

There would instantaneously be no more donations, no more jobs for those people, and no more money coming into that machine. An entire industry would become irrelevant overnight.

Now, if the cure happens to be something simple like (heaven forbid) proper nutrition, reduction of toxins in our food and air, a properly communicating nervous system without interference, decreased electrical waves in the form of WIFI, telephones, etc., and changing our lifestyles to reduce cellular mutations, well then my friends, that cure will be covered up faster than the crash site at Roswell. And it has been many times over.

This is the paradox of healthcare.

A cure in healthcare is a catastrophe because it is the death of an industry. What is more profitable is a partial cure in the form of a product (usually through a pill or needle) that only works while the individual is taking this product and has the added benefit of creating other problems in the body that need more partial cures to be taken long term.

This is why the only real things that are being heavily funded and researched are various forms of pharmaceutical drugs, aka partial cures. The goal of the corporations funding these drugs is to have you on medication that they supply you with from birth until death. And that's the reason the information from this book is so dangerous to the status quo and so necessary to find its way to the public. Especially now as this plan is reaching its epoch.

CHIROPRACTIC

I have been studying healthcare topics for over a decade through different careers and interests in the health and fitness field; however, my first in-depth experience of how far-reaching this paradox is came when I began my studies of medicine at a graduate level.

I was introduced to methods of medicine through the study of one of its biggest competitive modalities, Chiropractic.

Once I entered medicine through the backdoor, I made a point of looking around. Chiropractic school is comprehensive and includes extensive medical training in both the standard allopathic treatment protocols, as well as the reasoning and methods to view and treat dis-ease (the precursor to disease) through a Vitalistic viewpoint with the application of various chiropractic methodologies.

This was a huge eye-opener. It allowed me to compare notes and contrast opposing treatment protocols with how the body actually functions and the intended effects of each style of treatment to fix it. We were trained to look at the same situation and see the two different ways it could be understood and remedied and what those remedies would do for the individual's global health, both short and long-term.

An added and unexpected bonus to this compare-and-contrast training was that it provided me with a history lesson that revealed just how consistent and effective allopathic medicine has been at demonizing and destroying all inventions or practices of natural healing that threatened to interfere with the monopoly they have over the treatment of human health.

We have all heard the stories of the Witch Trials and of Zealots or Martyrs who have died for an idea that challenged current thought and authority (Jesus being the obvious first thought, however, not the only man or woman who fits that description). Surprisingly, this martyrdom does not exist solely in the religious realm. Many individuals died for attempting to challenge the commonly held beliefs regarding science as well. For example, how about when Galileo Galilei discovered that the earth revolved around the sun? This idea is now common knowledge, but what did he get for his brilliance and scientific discovery at the time? He was convicted of heresy by the church and sentenced to spend the rest of his life in house arrest, along with being forbidden to teach his discovery to anyone. Or what about the long-forgotten man named Giordano Bruno, who was burned at the stake for suggesting that the earth was in motion in the cosmos and not in a fixed place. Numerous companies and individuals have designed and created water-powered engines in the last century that have rivaled internal combustion engines in power, only to have their patents bought out and destroyed, never to be heard of again. Given that this could solve the entire climate change crisis worldwide, can you guess why these inventions have been so swiftly destroyed? Because you can get water from your sink, you don't have to buy it from a gas station after its cost has been inflated to line the pockets of the world's one percent.

The oil industry is a prime example of what happens when an industry gains total control over a field, like allopathic medicine has over human health, and how far they will go to keep it. So when Big Papa Joe, who flies everywhere in his private jet wearing six Rolexes on each arm, suddenly faces the possibility of having to give up one of them, Big Joe does whatever is necessary to make sure that doesn't happen. Even if that means destroying someone else's livelihood and hindering scientific progress. This is the pattern we see with all power and control over industry, and the pattern I learned that was very active in medicine.

When you start looking at the world we live in and why we are where we are as a civilization, you realize that money is the great motivator. The people who have it find a way to keep it, while the people who don't, claw tooth and nail to fight for the scraps.

Even though this aspect of life is universally known and generally, if not at least begrudgingly accepted, its ripple implications are not. You see, when we are all just working our asses off to get by, the most elusive but sought-after thing in the world is safety, security, and stability. This is a crutch that everyone wants to hold on to because they are already so overwhelmed that they can't handle any further stress and uncertainty. So when the very fabric of our society begins to crumble, and the foundational beliefs we have built our lives up begin to show obvious contradictions, most people begin to arm themselves with blinders and begin picking and choosing which aspects they can accept as corrupt based on their stress threshold, while doubling down on their conviction in the areas they cannot to avoid any added discomfort and uncertainty. The result of this is a population where everyone seems to have at least one political or ethical battle they have chosen to take a moral stand on while being oblivious to its interconnection with the larger machine of manipulation.

Think about it.

It's just like this big push to ban the use of plastic straws and now plastic bags. Is it not apparent to anyone else that this is the most ridiculous political fad designed only to make it look like governments are giving a shit about plastic production?

Think about how much plastic is in a single straw or bag…now think about how much plastic is used in a single pill bottle, or that came wrapped in the box you just ordered from Amazon, or around every single product you just bought from the grocery store but had to carry in your hands because you can no longer get a bag. Plastic straws and bags are such a tiny fragment that, yes, I agree a little is better than none, but do you see how many people are talking about this and fixated on it as some political heroism, all while completely ignoring the fact that absolutely nothing is being done to stop the plastic production industry in general? I mean, why don't they shut down the production of bottled water? Surely a colossal amount more plastic must be made to make a single bottle than a straw.

Well, it's because the bottled water industry has giants lobbying for it. The straw industry didn't stand a chance because it is not making billions for any powerhouses at the moment, so they are easy to choke off and make it look like a step in the right direction.

The sad truth is that decisions made in the political realm are never genuinely about the good of the people and never about the unbiased betterment of the planet; they are moves made in a giant game of chess based on who has paid the most and how can they package a move for profit to look like a move for ethics and moralism.

We live in a world where hierarchies of power and political funnels have existed for thousands of years before we were ever born. Unless a piece of information, invention, or even idea can fit through that political funnel without posing a threat to an existing ideology or the authority and dominion of the current groups in power, then that thing or idea is not only rejected but burned to the ground along with any and everyone who supported it.

This has created not only the paradox of medicine but also the framework to breed increasing safeguards through setting up individuals who can act as the authority and gatekeepers of information in every field, thus cementing the framework of thought and power in place. If you control the story, you control the people.

The information in the upcoming chapters results from these two distinct paradigms clashing (vitalistic/chiropractic vs. mechanistic/ allopathic), and the effects it is having on the world. I hope to shed light on the contrast between these two paradigms and summarize some of the most profound and powerful ideas about human health that I have come across in my studies over the past 14+ years.

I also will be presenting some original ideas that have developed within my own framework of understanding over the past several years that could change how we see human health forever...

These ideas, though original in my conception of them, have been birthed through the countless other ideas and theories I have encountered over the years in both formal and informal education. This information, as said before, is not a complete and exhaustive report of all of the truths available about human health, but it is intended to provide a starting point for both the average individual and the highly educated practitioner alike to integrate this new information into your own frameworks of belief about who and what you really are, and provide tools to take back the control of your own body and own health for the rest of your life.

Because I owe much of the framework of my understanding to the lens provided to me through the principles of chiropractic, it is also my intention to provide some background on the third most popular form of healthcare in the world behind allopathic medicine and dentistry and give you a quick rundown as to why the allopathic medical machine has worked so hard to destroy it.

CHAPTER 1

A CALL TO ACTION

We live in an unprecedented time in science, healthcare, and politics. We are seeing swaths of unrelenting and unapologetic methods of censorship, bias, and pseudoscientific ideas being implemented and dubbed as scientific facts while witnessing the systematic eradication of natural health practices and philosophies worldwide.

Though maybe at a higher scale now than before, this is nothing new. Politics and science have always been two distinct sides of the same coin. Both rule with an iron fist within their distinct domains and bulldoze every hint of competition or perceived heresy as they march the machine forward, while acquiring unthinkable amounts of money and gaining unimaginable control.

At the turn of the 1900s, humans entered an era of supposed agency and personal authority predicated on the scientific and industrial revolutions. After the Great Wars were fought and heinous crimes were committed, we passed out to the other side with a new sensation of relief and freedom, which was held up by a promise that nothing like that would ever happen again. The people of the world were told that from then on, we all had the right and freedom to choose what we believed, who we worshiped, and what we did to and with our bodies.

Born in the late 1980s, my generation grew up with an unquestioned sense that we were free to make our own choices, for better or worse. We had an open slate to decide who and what we were with only a few hard lines we knew we were not supposed to cross: Don't do drugs, don't steal, don't swear at your mom, say please and thank you, and don't cause physical violence upon anyone else. Outside of those main guides and our own unique parental influences, we were essentially free to do, say, and think whatever we wanted. Or at least so it seemed.

We are realizing now that even during those seemingly golden times, an evil machine was still moving in the background. The machine moved quietly and strategically, acquiring knowledge and power from the events and power transfers of the Great Wars to become an even more stealthy and dangerous entity, setting its sights on our future. Playing the slow game.

This silent machine became a covert force that ran in the shadows like a lion slowly stalking its prey. Since we didn't have the internet at the time, the news stations *seemed* to be much less biased, and people trusted them. We all lived in the comfort of the idea that we were being told the truth, the government cared about us, and the news told us all the facts about what was happening in the world and our communities. We knew that the hospitals and medicine as a whole were going to be there to save us if anything bad happened and that we were being watched out for by companies and policies set up to protect us and our way of life. This was a beautiful illusion and one that I miss dearly because it made life a whole lot more predictable.

There was comfortable security in the agreement to be a good person, work hard, and pay your taxes in exchange for the assurance that no one would get in your way or take advantage of you and that someone would always be there to help. If something happens to go wrong, don't worry; you will be taken care of.

You get what you give, quid pro quo.

Those were the good old days.

Like waking up abruptly from a dream, the eye-opening events of the last four years have stripped the layers away from that fantasy. From the coordinated response to the pandemic to the stripping of millions of people's rights and segregating people based on their decisions to remain in control of their bodily autonomy and medical choices, to the detrimental implementations of lockdowns worldwide, to a well-documented child pedophilia ring involving a staggering amount of powerful and influential people, to the coordinated destruction of thousands of food suppliers, to the fabricated recession, to coordinated and planned forest fires, to the total and complete censorship of news and information being let into supposedly sovereign democratic countries... We have seen the mask removed from the machine.

Piece by piece, we have seen basic and intrinsic truths about this world slowly become muddied, blurred, and then completely flipped upside down. We have witnessed the media lie, omit, and alter facts about current events on a scale so large and so obvious that it is hard to believe that we aren't living in some bizarro world prank.

Politics have hijacked medicine, and medical advice has become based only on political and private interests instead of scientific evidence. Medicine transitioned from evidence-led to politics-led. We have watched as medical advice transitioned from advice to forceful recommendations, to mandates, to the (overuse of this word)manipulation of information to convince the unknowing public of whatever ideologies were most useful at that time. We watched as free speech platforms censored and destroyed any person or idea that doesn't fit the agreed-upon narrative, even if that information is presented by highly esteemed and qualified individuals in their fields. The hidden machine has come out of hiding and begun demonstrating its reach in a way that has shaken the world.

The unsuspecting people of the world have watched this all happen in awe and disbelief.

As for myself, I should have been surprised; I should have been completely and utterly shocked as well. But I wasn't.

Instead, it seemed oddly familiar because this same method of censorship and propaganda has been used to disrupt and destroy every system of alternative medicine that has been developed that contradicts the agreed upon and elite-funded narrative of germ theory and pharmaceutical intervention for decades. I just so happened to have spent the last four years before these events studying this historical pattern, particularly in the one I chose to pursue as a profession. The only difference with the pandemic was that it was carried out using a much more aggressive campaign and on a much broader scale. Though none of the tactics they used surprised me, the part that did surprise me was how many people fell for it and still are to this day.

I am just grateful that I chose the career I did because it prepared me for what has happened and taught me what to look out for. Like a playbook given to the other team, little by little, I, and others like me, watched it unfold.

By deciding to become a chiropractor, I unsuspectingly stumbled into a profession that has been systematically attacked, censored, and stigmatized at the hands of mainstream medicine and its sponsors for the last 128 years. Like most people, I was oblivious to the fact that chiropractic was a sworn enemy of mainstream medicine when I chose to pursue it; however, once entering graduate studies and learning the well-documented history of attacks on chiropractic, I was outright infuriated that something that could help so many people was being systematically marginalized.

Though we are not the only natural healing modality to receive such special treatment in the last century, we are one of the most heavily and consistently smeared and contended. In the last four years, however, we have seen a level of censorship that has extended far past just our professions' walls and into all arenas of progressive scientific thought and natural health practices. This newly intensified campaign threatens not only the extinction of my profession but also the global access to natural health ideas and treatments for people in countries all around the world. In Canada specifically, it threatens even to limit our access to naturally derived vitamins, minerals, and health food products as early as 2025.

Witnessing this happen on such a grand scale right in front of my eyes, especially after studying it through the history of my profession, makes me feel like I am living through some strange combination of Ground Hog Day and George Orwell's 1985.

When faced with dire situations, we always have two choices: action or inaction.

Do something or do nothing.

I am the kind of person who never really considers the second option.

Given that, I felt it was an apt time to try and provide a source of information that I hope can serve as a tool of awakening, or more accurately, of *remembering* the truth of who and what we are, along with our natural ability to heal and break free from the chains and limiting beliefs that are holding us down.

Despite coordinated attempts to change our perception of ourselves, the truth can never be truly erased. We only lose the control we willingly give away. As long as the ideas remain, they can be passed on to others. Due to censorship pressures and increasing levels of content control, we are running out of time to reclaim our body sovereignty, and that starts with relearning how our bodies *actually* work and what is required to maintain them, for ourselves, and all our future generations.

With that in mind, let's begin.

THE INSUFFICIENCY OF MEDICAL KNOWLEDGE

As a species, humans are designed to adapt. The sensation of those adaptations and of the process of adapting, however, may be uncomfortable or feel strange or foreign if you do not know what to expect. Those sensations are then usually deemed as a disorder or symptom of illness. This is because we have not been taught that we are supposed to undergo these transitions or that they are natural and inevitable. Instead, these transitions have been turned to pathologies in our modern world, and therefore, our modern collective conscious psyche instantly deems them as bad, and we act accordingly to try and banish them.

Would a snake worry as the process of shedding its skin began if its internal instincts didn't know that it was not only beneficial but also inevitable? Would a dog begin to tremble as its hair started to come out in clumps as the winter months slowly turned to summer? What other species is met with anxiety as they witness their bodies undergoing natural transformations based on either seasonal changes or internal and external environmental changes? The answer to this question is, none.

We alone exist in this category.

Most of the anxieties that we feel as humans consist of the either the general fear of death, or the fears of bodily and mental dysfunction that have been trained into us since birth. But what if many of the things we consider to be dysfunctions were (overuse of word actually) natural and appropriate processes taking place inside our bodies and minds and we were just taught the wrong stories about them? What if we found out new stories that made much more sense and replaced the old ones? What then?

How would we see our symptoms? More importantly, how would we live differently knowing the new stories?

If we were given the knowledge of the *appropriate* and *natural* processes of our body, along with the natural abilities of our mind to interact with the matter around us, fear would cease to exist, and it would be replaced with sheer and utter amazement. Even more importantly, it would be replaced with confidence, personal security, and complete body awareness and autonomy. If we knew we were gods, we would have the confidence of gods.

If we were to understand the simple processes of our body and the way in which our bodies and minds work, then so many of the sensations we encounter that evoke such high levels of anxiety would disappear, and fear of hospital rooms and morgues would vanish. We would no longer need to project these terrible possibilities into our imaginations because we would no longer be stuck in the cycles of mortal fear spawned from our lack of self-assurance and self-knowledge. Instead, we would live in a place of total calmness, understanding the circle of life but knowing how resilient we are throughout it. But because of our lack of understanding, and through the intentional guidance of the medical giants, it is instead the inevitable deterioration of our body that plagues us most and which serves as the basis of almost all other forms of fear that we experience throughout our lives. Our inevitable demise and deterioration are the main source of our eternal anguish.

Though it is inevitable that one day we will transition out of this material body into something else, there are also many untruths we have accepted as part of this transition that have colored this inevitable change with the feelings of impending doom that seem to trouble us every single day. The human experience is a complex topic, but to attempt to understand it, I always return to the human body because that is the field in which I have been trained and am the most familiar. Through learning about ourselves, we learn about the world, but instead of embarking on this noble pursuit, we have been encouraged not to be bothered with it and instead leave it up to professionals who promise (scouts honor!) to have our best interests in mind.

The problem is that along the way, these professionals began taking bribes to prescribe drugs and procedures that are not in our best interest, and money has taken control of their prescription pads. We have become a generation dependent on often corrupt professionals to guide us. At the same time, we desperately grope around in the dark, becoming increasingly oblivious to the normal functions of this meat vehicle each of us is riding in.

DISSECTING THE PROBLEM

When a student begins any form of medical training, it's the mental equivalent of opening their mouth to a firehose and hoping to drink as much as possible. The amount of information they are exposed to can be rather overwhelming, to say the least. They spend years studying the details of the various systems of their body, along with all of their intertwined positive and negative feedback loops. It takes an immense amount of time and effort to get to a place where you can have a fairly basic sense of what is happening.

As you move higher in your training, you become more specialized. Getting down to the chemical and electrical level of any system requires a very powerful but narrow microscope of view, so the further specialized you become, the less you see or understand about the rest of the body as that old, unnecessary information drops out of your memory and focus. As you progress in your specialty, the base understanding you acquired in the earlier stage of your program seems to fade away as you focus your brain cells on the information relevant to your position.

Essentially, you begin to see the trees really damn well but have lost all sense of the forest. Sometimes, you can even spend an entire career focusing your microscopic vision on something that you eventually realize was a spec on the glass and tells you nothing about the specimen underneath. Imagine a mathematician studying a specific theorem. He spends years learning the intricacies of this theorem only to realize that it is built on assumed variables that must remain assumptions because no former mathematician has been able to prove them, nor can he, hence, why it remains a theory.

At this point, he realizes he can either continue to study and build on an assumption that has never been proven or abandon ship. Option two comes with the added sting of saying goodbye to his dreams of making a revolutionary breakthrough and admitting error. Given that option two requires starting from scratch and losing funding, tenure, and reputability, we can see why most would choose the first option and continue to perpetuate a story that no one truly knows if it is real or not.

There is nothing inherently wrong with the first option. I mean, who knows, maybe he can be the one to prove it and finally jump that theory forward. The problem isn't in the dedication to a field or the topic; the problem is that many things that have yet to be proven *are considered to be unquestionable facts*, and entire systems of procedures are already based on these assumptions.

Science and mathematics, when used appropriately and unbiasedly, are tools for understanding the divine and evolving our abilities as individuals and as a society. With these techniques, we have managed to develop incredible amounts of knowledge and technologies; however, despite only scratching the surface of what is possible with these tools, our collective egos have blinded us to the fact that the island of knowledge we sit on is just a piece of driftwood in the vast ocean of possibility.

A great example of this is the fact that we still don't understand the physiological processes of human consciousness or how we have the ability for someone like me to write and create completely novel thoughtforms and sentences in my mind using universally understood symbols and apply them to paper for others to immediately integrate into their world perceptions.

Though the idea of consciousness is considered to be the most complex of all human mysteries and functions, one could also argue that it is the most basic.

Our ability to consciously understand and interact with our environment and others within it at such a complex level is the basis of what makes us human and a distinct species. We have spent so much time focusing on perpetuating knowledge in the scientific realm that most people who are considered scientists do not even apply the scientific method themselves. Instead, most scientists and doctors are trained to perpetuate the ideas that are most agreed upon in our current time frame and seem to have given up the pursuit of some of the most basic but still unknown processes, like our consciousness. This means that we have more people repeating a story than trying to prove the story, and if you have any experience with our current social media frenzies, you can understand why that would be problematic. Parrots are rarely free-thinkers and seldom real scientists. But they can sure squawk loud.

To further demonstrate the point of assumed knowledge that has entire paradigms built on it but has never been proven is that we don't even know what a human cell *looks like* in its full capacity. We have supposed knowledge of all these structures that exist within it, including the nucleus, the nucleoli, the Golgi apparatus, and all other cellular structures that we are taught in cellular biology; however, we have no actual pictures of all of these structures existing within the cell that aren't computer generated best-guesses. The shapes of the structures we so surely teach on a daily basis to children and university students alike are not derived from actual pictures of these structures, but instead, they are scientific estimations using computer-generated CGI. We do not have any pictures or evidence that this is what a cell looks like inside—we do not have the technology to obtain such images. To fill in the technological gap, those images have been made through illustrations based on assumptions of perpetuated and accepted knowledge. Filling the gap with best guesses isn't the concern; after all, that is what is required in science until something is provable; however, it is the teaching of an unproven idea as unquestionable fact and building entire scientific and medical procedures on them.

If we do not actually know what a human cell looks like inside or understand how we exist in a conscious state, how are we supposed to have a real understanding of what the human body is? These are the two base starting points for understanding human existence. One represents the mental, and the other represents the physical. If we do not truly know how these two base starting points work, how much more about our bodily functions are based on guesstimations? If we are building on two shoddy foundations, how stable are the structures we are creating?

When you really get down to it, the supposed masters of the field of medicine are so unnervingly unaware of the actual structures and functions of the human body it's shocking.

Despite our personal feelings about this, this is the truth. As unsettling as it may be, I like to think that in some ways, it is also amazingly comforting.

When you realize that all of the physical limitations that have been placed on our bodies and minds from scientific and medical wisdom are just ideas based on assumptions and best guesses, then the door to other possibilities and opportunities opens.

Do you want to go through it?

BE FOR SOMETHING, NOT AGAINST SOMETHING

It is important for me to get the point across that this book and the information within it is neither intended to be *anti*-medicine nor *anti*-establishment; instead, it is meant to be *pro*-empowerment and *pro*-human. It was written for one purpose: to educate the public about their own bodies. I hope to make it clear how and why it is important for you to understand yourself on this level and why now, more than ever, it is imperative that you take responsibility for your own health.

If you don't, no one else will.

I also hope that the insights and perspectives within can refocus laypeople and medical practitioners of all kinds to strive to celebrate and work *with* the body and not *against* it.

In our current state of information overload—and *mis*information overload—we, as consumers and humans, are more confused than ever. This is hardly our fault, however, because, as mentioned, not only are we being constantly bombarded with contradictory and incorrect information, but it is also easier than ever to spread an idea (whether true or not) simply by having influence and exposure on social media, paid for news stations, or just deeply lined pockets.

Pay attention next time you hear someone debating politics or posting constructed pictures about anti-vaxxers, flat-earthers, or any other collectively decided antagonist of the time. If you look carefully, you will see that the phrases they are using and the verbiage they choose are phrases and verbiage programmed into them by someone or somewhere else. Even the term anti-vaxxers or flat-earthers is a purposeful naming of a group with degrading connotations attached to it to lower that group's credibility subconsciously. Anytime a person has a belief or idea that falls into one of these pre-named categories, they are slapped with the accompanying label, along with the ever-popular title of "conspiracy theorist." This instantly robs them of credibility and persuades the unknowing public to disregard anything they say before they are fully heard. (Fun fact: the term conspiracy theorist was created by the CIA after the assassination of President John F. Kennedy to discredit the individuals who were claiming it was an inside job).

The worst thing about these terms is that they are perpetuated by herd mentality. Studies have shown people would rather be wrong than disliked. No one wants to be associated with anyone who is placed in a socially condemned category unless they have firm enough beliefs to handle the social exile that comes with it.

Just jump on your Facebook feed, and it won't take long to see a picture being shared with information that contradicts the current narrative, accompanied by a fact-check notification below it. This is done on purpose to not only degrade all possible forms of dangerous and powerful anti-establishment movements but also to keep us divided. It is much easier to keep us confused and under control when we are distracted and separated. And for anyone who is sitting in the middle on any topic, the notice of a post being fact-checked serves as the subconscious red light that makes them decide to place their belief on the safe and socially supported side of the fence.

The reason I bring these examples up is not to blur the story or take away from the point of this book in any way; rather, it is intended to simply point out the fact that when we begin to discuss the topic of medicine, we need to realize that it is only a single part in a very well-oiled and very powerful collective machine that has all of the aforementioned safeguards instilled within it. It is a single branch on a tree of political and human control using a confusion-for-profit campaign. As we go forward, remember that nothing in politics is ever completely isolated, nothing in politics is free from policies of profit, and nothing in medicine is free from either.

* * *

When it comes to where you stand on any topic, you can choose one of two ways to approach it: You can either be *for* something, meaning you hold beliefs and take actions to support and spread an idea or thing, or you can be *against* something, in which your goal, ideas, and actions are about trying to stop something. This is an important distinction to make for yourself on any topic of interest because it will help you decide where you want to focus your energy and where you don't. For me, being *against* something has a negative energy about it — a destructive and disruptive energy. It is usually associated with trying to stick it to the man and protest something you believe is wrongfully acting upon either yourself, a specified group, or society as a whole. Though this form of energy is useful, and I am all for sticking it to the man when he is being an asshole, that is not the energy I want to use to spread the information in this book.

The energy I would like to surround the information in this book with comes instead from a place of love, optimism, and hope. Being *for* something has a very positive energy attached to it, which is my conscious intention for this information. How something makes you feel is often more important than what that thing is, says, or does. Being for something is constructive. It's about creating and perpetuating a frequency and an idea because you believe in and care about it.

It's about *creation,* not destruction.

It's about risking everything because you support a cause or idea and realize that it is greater than you. I want this book and my career to be about that.

I also want you to be empowered to see yourself and the world around you with a different lens — one that will excite you and expand your idea of just how much you are capable of. Using ancient philosophy, esoteric wisdom, and modern scientific thought, I hope to demonstrate to you that we are much more powerful than we have been told.

I hope to show you yourself in a way you may have never seen. I hope to show you the other side of human health and function—the one that isn't taught to us through the mainstream channels because it is a threat to the priests and cardinals of the newest and most powerful world religion: The Religion of Science.

CHAPTER 2

THE RELIGION OF SCIENCE

In the last few decades, there has been a steep decline in interest in organized religion, being replaced by an increase in the number of people who are blindly throwing their faith in science to fill the void. Unfortunately, despite this seemingly rational decision by many, blind and unquestioning belief in science is just as dangerous as blind and unquestioning belief in religion; only this version is based on the flawed premise that science is worthy of this faith because it is unbiased, "real," and uncensored.

Unfortunately, this couldn't be further from the truth.

Outside of the fact that the empirical method is fundamentally limited by only being able to prove linear actions and effects within controlled and un-realistic environments (a luxury we do not have when considering the real functions of the human body, or the world for that matter), the scientific method also has another huge, gaping flaw:

To conduct and publish a scientific study that is going to be taken seriously takes money. Lots of it.

You can't simply design any experiment you want and just go out and do it – at least not one that will reach further than your bedroom. Studies require resources to bring them to fruition. *Lots* of resources. Time, money, manpower, controlled environments, statisticians, volunteers, credible authors and institutions to back them, etc. All these elements are needed even to begin a properly crafted study, let alone see it to completion and attempt to have the results published.

Not only do you have to pay for the physical tools required, i.e., the electricity, the building in which you conduct the study, the usage of the tools or specialty devices used to record the findings, the cost of the materials required, and on and on. You also have to pay the wages of every person who is working on these projects, including the test subjects, all while being able to promote the study enough to get it considered for peer reviewing and publication once countless hours have been spent sifting through the data to determine its statistical significance, if any.

None of that is cheap. So why is this a problem?

Well, do you actually think anyone would be willing to pay for all that without the promise or at least the high likelihood of a large return on their investment? Everything is business, and this is business 101. Do not invest in something if the expected return on investment is less than the cost of the investment. And let's face it; there aren't many billionaires with hearts so big they are willing to shell out wads of cash just for the good of science and the betterment of human health. And the ones who pretend they are … Well, we all know how that is currently working out for us.

Unbiased scientific studies are, at the very best, hard to come by and, at the worst, non-existent. If the result of a study or experiment paid for by an investing group happens to show a conclusion that none of the parties funding it can make a profit from, the results of that study are either buried, erased, or highly doctored to create an illusion of success. The original idea, however, along with the chance of further research into that idea, are either abandoned or shifted to another line of research that has a higher likelihood of profitability. This means that study results that are good for humanity but not good for profitability tend to vanish into the ether.

Knowing this, we can see how the evolution of the scientific machine has systematically hijacked true, altruistic scientific investigation, replacing it with a highly powerful tool used almost exclusively to fund validation for products and treatments owned and exploited for profit. Despite the honest and genuine humans out there pursuing all things good for the world, this is the unfortunate reality we find ourselves in.

* * *

The scientific pursuit started as a practice of the empirical method to gain an understanding of the world we live in. It was intended to be based on the pure and noble search for the demonstrable truth. Unfortunately, this unadulterated and noble pursuit became monopolized and monetized almost immediately as it became recognized as a powerful tool of control. The pursuit of the big questions of who and why we are what we are slowly became muddied and shifted into a well-designed machine that could serve as a tool to create a level of mass obedience never before imagined and make those in power more powerful and those who aren't, quiet, mystified, powerless, and ignorant.

Most people living today hold science as the unquestioning authority without knowing almost anything about it or the money that drives it. People who talk the most about trusting science have the least understanding of what genuine science is. After all, "trust the science" is probably the most anti-science statement ever made.

Even the individuals who complete an undergraduate degree and consider themselves educated in scientific fields most often don't know the current state of that field at its upper levels. Undergraduate degrees serve more as a brief history of accepted dogma. They teach you enough to passionately perpetuate your field's antiquated and politically endorsed ideas. It isn't until graduate school that most people start actually pursuing their original thoughts and ideas, only to find that the higher they go in their education, the less certainty they find, until eventually they reach the apex of their field and find all of the highest minds around them frantically arguing about the validity of some of the most basic assumptions you learned in your first years. This leads to the anxiety-ridden realization that *the true experts are actually confused as fuck.*

But spoiler alert: that's how science is supposed to be!

Scientific advancement can only happen when differing ideas are contested, and brilliant minds spend their entire careers trying to prove themselves right and their competition wrong. Consensus has never brought innovation, and "trusting the science" has never been a tenant of science.

Why would it be?

Old Man Einstein had it right: the more you know, the more you know you don't know. Any individual who is dead set on their unshakable beliefs in a particular field of science has likely either not studied it for long enough, not investigated it at all, is arguing for their own idea, or is being paid very well to stand so firmly.

Everyone is searching for the elusive Theory of Everything, but it has yet to be discovered. Knowing that, by definition, no theory or branch of knowledge about the human body or human experience, or the universe itself for that matter, answers all questions and variables simultaneously and is all-inclusive and all-encompassing. This also means that no theory or field of scientific knowledge is or ever will be unquestionable. Period.

All branches of science have at their very backbone a series of set assumptions that have not been fully proven, as we often don't have the means or technology to be able to prove many of them, or we often decide we trust the assumptions so much that they aren't worth proving at all. Despite being unproven or unprovable, they have nevertheless formed the underlying accepted dogma of each field and serve as the seemingly stable foundation for all other beliefs and research to be built upon pertaining to that topic.

The smartest minds in every field know this to be true and know this to be the nature of science, but it's the newbies and the non-sciencey folk that don't. The greatest minds in any generation are those who know that life is full of unknowns and that our limits of experience mean that life is lived in gray areas. And when it comes to knowledge about the human body and human experience, *there are nothing but gray areas.*

CHAPTER 3

THE RELIGION OF SCIENCE, IN MEDICINE

If science is the religion, then medical doctors are the priests, rabbis, and the Holy men and women. In the Western world, few hold a higher social rank and demand higher respect than a medical doctor, but let's examine this for a second and see if this status and veneration is rightfully placed or if it is just an antiquated idea we unnecessarily adhere to as the status quo. After all, everyone wants their kid to grow up to be a doctor, right?

I want to be clear that I truly believe there are thousands of genuinely skilled, good-intentioned, highly trained, lifesaving medical practitioners out there who spend their entire lives helping anyone who needs it. I applaud and respect the shit out of them, and they save hundreds of thousands of lives across the world every single day. No one can or will ever diminish that, and for those actions, we as a society are incredibly lucky to have them. So first, let's look at the reasons medical doctors *do* deserve our admiration and appreciation.

If you have ever been in a bad car accident, found a relative collapsed on the floor, cut your finger off with a saw, snagged your thigh against a long rusty nail hanging out of a door jam, or come down with a severe case of pneumonia, food poisoning, infection, or any other medical emergency, you would have experienced the skilled help of one of these highly trained individuals. In fact, these people and the medical interventions they provide are likely the reason you or a loved one is still here today.

Medical doctors shine when dealing with emergency medical situations. The invention of antibiotics and the development of the practice of various surgical interventions have been some of the greatest lifesaving advancements in human history (a lot better now than a hundred years ago when they would just saw off your leg if it was infected). Of all areas of medicine, trauma surgery is probably the most impressive and consistently awe-inspiring. The fact that an individual can get a metal rod driven straight through their skull and somehow still live (every psychology student will be familiar with this case) is an absolutely mind-blowing achievement. Alongside trauma surgery, the fact that you can have a bum heart or kidney, and a surgeon can take one from someone else and replace it like a car part is undeniably incredible.

These achievements and countless more, demonstrate the true value and importance of the allopathic medical model. It is undisputed that when it comes to emergency care and emergency illness situations, allopathic medicine is absolutely the best choice, and the doctors and nurses who handle these cases every single day deserve our highest level of gratitude and respect. So if your son or daughter grows up to be a medical doctor, yes, you should be really damn proud.

But what happens when the person who receives the heart transplant begins to have memories and develops personality traits and mannerisms that aren't theirs but are those of the individual from whom they received the heart? Or when we have a growing epidemic of lifestyle-related diseases that are being treated with pills instead of changing the lifestyle that created them? Or when we have a statistically significant climb in childhood-related diseases, neurological disorders, and autoimmune disorders that are rising at the same rate as the increase in medication and vaccinations prescribed across the Western world? In the face of these dilemmas, allopathic medicine has proven to be a lot less of the all-knowing savior and a lot more like one of the three blind mice.

You see, despite allopathic medicine being an amazing practice for emergency injury and illness management, it is rather terrible at addressing risk management, long-term health, wellness, nutrition, mental health, biomechanics, and non-pharmacological interventions, while somehow managing to be almost oblivious to the universal fact that breaking the natural rules of the body can never lead to long-term health and should be left as the absolute last resort. Every pill takes from one side of the scale to add to another, and this is a balancing act that rarely results in positive, long-term health outcomes.

Now, I know what you are thinking: How am I possibly going to claim that allopathic medicine doesn't understand the natural effects of the body? They are supposed to be the *experts* on that, aren't they?

Well, they are *supposed* to be. However, because of the lens through which they are trained to see the body, medical doctors are often left staring at a single branch of a tree while missing the entirety of the forest, to use this analogy again. Sometimes, it seems, they don't even know they are in a forest.

CHOOSE YOUR LENS CAREFULLY

In allopathic or Western medicine, the body is treated much the same as a machine. Each part of a machine can be isolated to its specific function and can exist independently of the whole. By applying this same simplified logic to the human body, you end up with a paradigm that acts as if each system, organ, or function of the body can be isolated and treated without that treatment affecting any other system, organ, or function. This is called the Mechanistic model of Health, and it forms a specific lens through which all individuals trained in this model look to see and evaluate health.

Through this lens, if you have high blood pressure, it is believed that you can treat it by artificially lowering the blood pressure with chemical agents, aka pharmaceuticals, as a first line of defense. It is also believed that these chemical agents will not have any negative effects on other areas of your health; however, if you happen to be "unlucky," and they do, then you can add another chemical agent to counteract it. Ironically, despite wreaking havoc on any other body system or how many "unlucky" side effects you experience, if these pharmaceuticals do lower your blood pressure, they are considered a success and recommended for long-term use. All the other side effects along the way can simply be treated by adding another pharmaceutical to the mix. Take from one side of the scale, add to the other, and hope that you can find a balance. Simple as that.

Despite this method having a nearly non-existent cure rate and a very well-known pattern of health decline with every additional medication added to the routine of each patient, this is the exclusive treatment path for nearly all conditions in the Western world, regardless of their cause or association with lifestyle or dietary problems.

This approach has become so accepted because it has full endorsement by medical professionals; the reason those medical professionals endorse it is because it is based on the most prevalent medical science.

But why is that?

Why does it so happen that almost all medical science conducted around the world involves prescribing some chemical agent or another? Because a chemical intervention can be created and patented, and researching the effects of a single chemical agent fits very well into the standards of double-blind studies, which are regarded as the gold standard in scientific research and has led to a very real bias in what is considered a good study or a bad study.

A double-blind study looks for a one-to-one relationship in which a single research parameter can be affected by a single experimental factor. In the blood pressure case above, administering an Ace Inhibitor or Beta Blocker would result in a statistically significant lowering of the blood pressure in the study being conducted. If this is the case, and it can be repeated over multiple subjects, then they label the drug as a success and begin putting a price tag on it. (This is a slightly simplified explanation. The true process would involve progressing to second and third-stage trials; however, in certain high-profile scenarios, such as the rushed process to release an experimental genetic modification in 2021, this process can be modified, shortened, or bypassed altogether if enough money is thrown at it).

So, what's wrong with this lens?

Let's take a step back and use a different one to view this situation. Let's use a more holistic lens of health, which views the body as a single whole, intimately interconnected and inseparable in all ways. More specifically, let's use the *chiropractic* lens.

ABOVE>DOWN, INSIDE>OUT

First and foremost, if you have high blood pressure, there is a reason. Blood pressure is affected by a multitude of factors in your body and environment, including things like altitude, emotions, climate, other medications, alcohol use, inflammation, stress, and the foods you eat, to name a few. So, if you have elevated blood pressure, it will be related to one or multiple definite causes within your body; it doesn't just elevate because it was bored or because your body was running low on Ace Inhibitors.

If someone presents with high blood pressure in my clinic, the first step would be to look for the *cause* of the high blood pressure. If it is chronically elevated, differentiating between possible causes of chronically high blood pressure, such as elevated stress levels, chronic systemic inflammation, weight, or a misalignment in your spine causing chronic overstimulation of your sympathetic nervous system, etc., would be a great place to start, and necessary if we want to actually find the cause and work to correct it naturally.

When looking at these possible reasons, we have to use the holistic lens to consider each one's specific physiological impacts, across all categories above and beyond just blood pressure. This will help us narrow down the options and help us use the patient's other health history as a resource for deepening our understanding of how and why we are seeing this problem. After this, we will need to maintain this lens when crafting the best approach to *correcting* the problem in the same multifaceted way.

Is it a chemical problem? (imbalance of electrolytes and potassium/ sodium balance, magnesium deficiency, too much calcium in your blood, or inflammation due to toxic overload, etc.) Is it a hormonal problem? (chronically elevated cortisol from stress within the body or your life, which also makes this partly an emotional/psychological problem and leads to imbalances in hormonal levels, such as testosterone/estrogen balance), or thyroid hormones, which may also be partly a chemical problem since lack of iodine is a key factor in many thyroid-related disorders); or is it a physical problem? (global systemic inflammation or spinal subluxation/misalignment creating an internal stress response and the release of calcitonin from your bones, which stimulates epinephrine production). This summary is just a simplified set of possible factors that need to be considered when looking at the *cause* of something like elevated blood pressure.

But do you want to guess how many of these factors, on average, a general medical practitioner investigates or asks about before providing a chemical agent to treat high blood pressure?

None.

Outside of commenting on whether an individual is too fat or smokes, there is practically zero consideration as to the cause of this condition, just the quick draw of the pen to the prescription pad.

WHICH LENS DO YOU PREFER?

How you or your medical practitioners interpret data, symptoms, and prognosis all comes down to the lens each individual looks through that will color their perception of the human body and dictate how they treat it. The allopathic medical lens is based on a mechanistic and chemical approach. The tools of this approach are prescription pills, injections, and surgery. Despite the limitations and shortcomings of these methods, these shortcomings are of no fault to the current medical doctors in practice, who earnestly do their absolute best to help their patients day in and day out. Instead, the more upsetting truth is that this is all by conscious design of the medical programs and institutions that taught them, which have been crafted to fuel the pharmaceutical industries and create a perceived barrier between humans and health, with medically trained individuals acting as the intermediary. Much like priests were designed to behave as the intermediaries between humans and God, doctors are designed to be the necessary intermediary between humans and health.

It's all designed to establish and maintain power.

As stated earlier in this chapter, the scientific method only works when you isolate variables and focus on specific target outcomes in unnaturally controlled environments. This means that all treatments considered evidence-based and scientifically sound have to be based on experimental models in which an artificial environment is created to limit as many confounding variables as possible, and evaluation of the outcome is limited to evaluating a single variable at a time.

But let me ask you this: have you ever gone to the doctor and had blood work done? You know that sheet they give you, right? The one with 100 different boxes with scientific words and coding written beside them… Well, it's likely that your sheet, once given to you by the doctor, only had a small percentage of those boxes checked. That means that during this bloodwork analysis, the lab technicians will only evaluate a small percentage of the possible different markers in your blood. They won't look at any of the other 100 or so possible markers. You could have off-the-chart abnormal readings in 30 other categories, but if they are not a category that was checked off, then a doctor would never detect them because nobody was looking at them for the purpose of that evaluation.

This is the fundamental flaw of medical science. And *this* summarizes exactly what the empirical method has always done and is designed to do. It is a selective microscopic lens that only looks where it is told to look and is incapable of evaluating multiple parameters at once.

The problem?

When you spend your entire life looking through a microscope, eventually, you forget what the real world looks like. Eventually, you begin to trick yourself into thinking that humans are exactly like the sterile single-use test tubes and pipettes used in the lab.

Too much time spent imagining and creating unnatural environments tends to lead to the belief in functions and treatments that are equally unnatural. It seems the further we have progressed in medical science, the more unnatural our views of health have become.

CHAPTER 4

THE OCCULT UNDERSTANDING OF THE HUMAN BODY

To shine a brighter light on the views that will be presented in this book, it is important first to take a look into the history of the healing profession which acts as the foundation I stand upon, as well as take a tour through some of the philosophies that were fundamental in helping me mold my understandings of the human body.

For the first stop on this tour, we will take a brief look at the profound and hidden history of chiropractic, and how some of the tactics used to discredit this natural healing practice closely mirror the tactics we are currently seeing on a global scale to oppress and discredit natural healing practices of all types.

Same playbook, wider net.

First, let's define a few terms that are relevant to this topic and the information herein.

When something is referred to as esoteric, it means it is "designed to be understood by the specially initiated alone," according to Webster's Dictionary definition. By comparison, the term occult simply means hidden. So, when we are talking about the occult and esoteric connections to the history of chiropractic, we are referring to the hidden knowledge and connections that are likely only to be understood by the few. This concept has been the basis of all mystery schools since the beginning of recorded history, including the Brotherhood of Freemasonry, The Rosicrucian Society, The Skull and Bones, The Royal Society, The Templar Knights, and so on.

To be a Freemason is a highly misunderstood but incredibly mysterious thing to most people outside of the lodge. How would I know? Well because I was outside the lodge looking in for many years before I was initiated as a third-degree Master Mason in 2020. Though I still do not truly know how I feel about the craft as a whole, or the life-long practice of it, versus life-long dedication to other religious and academic groups and practices, it was an experience I am incredibly grateful for and one that I believe to be fundamental in providing the insight and understanding that has allowed me to become the person I am today.

I began my journey into the lodge while studying in California and was raised to a third-degree Master Mason in my home country of Canada with the help of brother, as well as my close friend and sponsor, who introduced me to the lodge in California. There is much speculation and rumors about Freemasonry, but nobody really knows anything about the Masons except someone who has gone through the rites and rituals to become one. One rule of the lodge is no member can ever be solicited or scouted, so one must only join of their free will and accord and if they have taken the necessary steps to seek admission.

This means if you want to become a member, you need to find one and ask them to bring you in. There is no other way, and this is easier said than done.

Once introduced and invited into the lodge, the process is long (not as long as it used to be in years past; it wasn't uncommon to take anywhere from three to ten years to go from a first-degree to a third-degree), taking between one to three years in modern times. It took me roughly a year and a half to move from Entered Apprentice to Master Mason.

During this time, you must go through each degree consecutively, and in between each, you are tasked to memorize words and paragraphs from rituals of significance, along with lessons that are deemed of high importance for your spiritual growth and understanding of the craft. The process and rituals cannot be repeated here, or anywhere for that matter, as that is part of the sacred code and oath as a brother. However, unlike many would have you believe, not all of what goes on in a masonic lodge is secret; rather, secrecy is a tool necessary to make sure that individuals advance in their spiritual understanding at an appropriate speed and in a way that the individual can properly understand. This goes back to the saying, "You don't cast pearls before swine." There is no benefit to communicating more information than an individual is ready to receive.

Ancient and important knowledge over thousands of years has followed this pattern of procession and has been passed on in very similar fashions within all mystery schools. Truths are taught and passed on through veiled and coded rituals and rites, never written in plain English (or any written language) so as to never allow them to fall into the wrong hands and be taken in by the untrained and unprepared mind. The information bestowed on the individuals who earn the opportunity to hear it is always layered and multifaceted but usually has some reference to the human body as a codex for each mystery. You see, within the mystery schools of human history, the human body is the most sacred and fundamental of all forms of spiritual and intellectual endeavors. It is said that if you truly understand the human body, you understand all of the cosmos and everything within them. Because of this profound connection to the human body and the human experience as a whole, admission to one of these mystery schools in the past was not only sought after by the greatest minds in history but was usually a prerequisite to their success and world-changing discoveries. This is how things were in the founder of chiropractic, D.D. Palmer's times, back in the late 1800s and early 1900s, and this is exactly why the founder, his son, and the majority of the first Chiropractic schools in history were all members of the Masonic Brotherhood. In fact, many of the first schools were held in Masonic halls.

Today, the essence of the mystery schools, such as Freemasonry, remains to some small extent; however, there have been many masons who have left the lodge or broken the rules and decided to share the information they were taught for one reason or another. Fortunately, or unfortunately, I can't quite figure out which one — the concern about the information falling into uninitiated and dangerous hands really isn't as much of a concern as it may have once been. As it turns out, having the appropriate mental and spiritual preparation to receive this sacred knowledge seems to be fundamental in the ability to take it seriously and actually understand the complexity and implications of the information anyways. So, despite the effort to keep this information safe, a lot of the principles and teachings have been distributed amongst non-members over the last few decades. Unfortunately for the world, only a very small percentage of that information has been understood, and even less has been practically applied to increase human health and better the whole of humanity.

Instead, the availability of the information inside these mystery schools to the public has only led to further confusion, demonization, and assumptions about not just masonry but all forms of esoteric and occult knowledge. Despite this and the negative connotations around the topic of occult and esoteric information, I believe this area of study is fundamental in developing a true and robust understanding of the human body and human experience. It is my hope that for at least a small portion of that sacred knowledge, this book will serve as its own version of a codex to help you integrate this knowledge in a practical and applicable way.[2]

---

[2] If at the end of this book you find yourself having a greater interest in the esoteric understandings of the human body, then I would highly recommend reading "Man: The Symbol of the Great Mysteries" by Manly P. Hall, as well as the rest of his published work and recorded audio lectures, as he is the undisputed authority in esoteric writing, and a 33rd degree mason.

CHAPTER 5

KNOW THYSELF

"To know thyself is the beginning of wisdom"
- Socrates

As stated in the previous chapter, the ancient teachings of the mystery schools considered the human body to be not only the most sacred of all things but also the living codex to understanding the divine, God, and the cosmos.

When you begin to understand the human body and the hidden mysteries within our make-up, you begin to better understand the hidden mysteries in our reality. We are a miraculous interconnection of trillions of individual cells that all work independently, each having an incredible array of individual processes and structures inside of them all functioning on their own, but also somehow working together to keep each cell alive. The cells then work independently and cohesively to keep the tissue they exist within alive, as the tissues also work to keep the organs and systems they contribute to alive, and they all work together simultaneously to keep the body alive. While this is all happening, the body somehow has a conscious perception of only a tiny fraction of the processes taking place within it at any given moment but is somehow able to perceive and interpret the world outside of it and is able to think about any abstract idea it wants to while possessing the ability to create and make changes in the physical world at will to bring those ideas to life.

Excuse me, but that is fucking *insane.*

Even more insane is the fact that we have an estimated three times more bacteria inside us and on our outer skinsuit than the number of our own cells, and those bacteria are fundamental in not only keeping us alive, protected, and functioning properly but also play a role in our mental and perceptual states to a degree that modern science is only just beginning to be aware of.

We consist of not only our own cells but trillions of other cells that are independent of us but depend on us for them to exist, and they all work together in a beautiful symphony to create and maintain each of us in existence. We are a standalone community of human and non-human cells that work as a cohesive team to maintain our independent physical and conscious existence.

We are an entire universe unto ourselves, and just like our individual cells, we exist and function independently to create our own realities while being intrinsically linked with every other person around us to create, maintain, and sustain the collective reality.

This is the basis and backbone of all mystery school teachings. All ancient esoteric texts. All occult systems. Their foundation is the understanding that *we are the most powerful entities in our existence because our existence is based on our perception, and we are the forces that, whether we know it or not, create it and change it at will.*

We have the power to change our reality any time we want. If our perception *is* our reality, and we have the full ability to change our perception, then we have the literal power to change reality for ourselves whenever we decide. You are created but also a creator. You have the divine ability of will and opportunity right in your very hands, and you always have. Now, can you feel that? That is the *knowing* inside of you. That's the feeling you get when a truth that you have always known deep down to your core is being revealed to you. That is the remembering of your divine self.

Almost all self-help books, including and especially the movement of the book *The Secret,* have borrowed from this esoteric information and attempted to water it down and mass produce it to present extremely simplified versions of this occult wisdom in a way that could be easily digestible by the masses while being presented as an original idea.

There is power here, in this wisdom, beyond what you could imagine, and that is why this information has been considered so sacred and so important for thousands of years that many people over many centuries have been willing to die to keep it safe. Mystery schools have guarded, shaped, and perpetuated this information for thousands of years to maintain it in existence so it could one day be used to liberate humanity as a whole from the mental and spiritual slavery that we have been placed under since the dawn of time. The greatest minds in history have been members of these groups and have used these teachings on countless occasions to further understand their areas of expertise, often even giving credit to these schools for their discoveries that have shaped and molded humanity along the way.

Almost every influential scientist in history that we have learned about in countless textbooks has been either a hobbyist, or dedicated occultists and members of at least one of these mystery schools. Unfortunately, this information isn't printed in our textbooks but is nevertheless just as true as any of the lasting work from these scientists that has stood the test of time and shaped our modern lives. Below are just a few examples, but keep in mind that an entire encyclopedia could be written on this topic alone.

Do you remember the Pythagorean theorem? The one we were taught in grade school. You know, A squared plus B squared equals C squared?

$$a^2 + b^2 = c^2$$

Everyone remembers being taught this equation as the way to find the hypotenuse of a triangle, but interestingly, no one knows anything else about Pythagoras, the man who created it. Like the fact that he was single-handedly one of the most influential occultists of all time and the highest-ranking member of the mystery schools of his day.

Pythagoras has gone down as one of the most influential thinkers, scientists, and philosophers ever to walk this earth, yet he never wrote a single book or treatise himself. His accomplishments and interests were vast, and he was even said to be the inventor of musical notes and scales based on his finding that if he cut a string in exactly half, its note would be the same as the previous longer string but would be one octave higher, and vice versa. On top of inventing the musical scale, he is also dubbed to be the father of both geometry and numerology as a practice. Along with all his impressive accomplishments, he also had his very own philosophical school. For one to join and learn from him, they had to first show their commitment to the path of truth by *not speaking a single word* for five years before they could be considered for entry. Do you remember that scene from Fight Club where Bob waits on the porch for five days to pass the initiation rights and become a member of Project Mayhem?

Yeah, something like that. Except for five years!

Five years of silence just to be *initiated* into his teachings! If that doesn't scream mystery school, I don't know what does! What I would give to be a fly on the wall inside their meetings and hear what was being discussed.

Another more recent example that may be a bit more familiar is a man who you likely will recognize for his most famous works but may be completely amazed when you find out the details of the rest of his studies. I am speaking about none other than the famous Sir Isaac Newton.

You remember Isaac Newton, right? You know, the guy we mentioned in the last chapter? The father of Newtonian physics? The creator of the laws of thermodynamics? The literal foundation of the mechanistic and material paradigm of thought that we use to predict and measure the rules of our physical reality? Well, Newton was not only a member of multiple mystery schools during his life, as well as an obsessive and accomplished alchemist, but also potentially one of the greatest occultists that has ever lived, and he saw the world as *anything but* mechanistic.

It has been discovered since his death that Newton wrote more papers and manuscripts on alchemy and occult ideas than he ever wrote on principles of physics. Those manuscripts have been hidden from the world, and this portion of his life and insights from one of the greatest minds in history have been systematically deleted from the mainstream story.

Why?

Because you can't use someone as the face of the very useful theory of a mechanistic reality when he spent more time researching the unseen and spiritual aspects of reality than he ever spent under a tree getting barraged by falling apples.

The editing and cherry-picking of the life and history of Isaac Newton is a prime example of an individual who has been used as the face of an idea and agenda that wasn't theirs. Newton, and so many like him, perhaps even Jesus, have had their life's work and story obscured over time to eventually create a myth that does not accurately portray them or their true intentions. In Newton's case, his own work was used to discredit and defame one of his greatest interests and passions. Still to this day, Newton is used as the basis for discrediting all forms of occult, esoteric, and "pseudoscientific" lines of scientific investigation despite those exact types of investigations being the foundation from which the mechanistic principles were derived.

I have used these examples not only because they are interesting but also to demonstrate my point that all scientific thought can be linked back to esoteric wisdom, even the most seemingly mechanistic and basic ideas.

The principles and beliefs of chiropractic were crafted using similar wisdom; the only difference is that chiropractic originally embraced these origins publicly in the formation of their 33 guiding principles instead of shamefully hiding their connections. The chiropractic principles are a set of truths about reality and the human body that were taken from the same common sources as the ideas that have inspired and influenced the greatest minds in scientific history. Despite the significance of this connection, when spoken about today, instead of providing credibility and legitimacy to our practice by showing direct lineage to the wisdom that has changed our world throughout the ages, it invokes ridicule, mistrust, and criticism.

This connection leads scientifically trained individuals and lay people alike to make false assumptions about the legitimacy and scientific foundation of the practice of chiropractic, regardless of how effective its treatments have proven to be.

The thing that most people do not know, however, and what most scientists are unwilling to admit, is that all science and scientific breakthroughs have a firm connection with the occult and the teachings of the mystery schools because these are *the origins of all scientific understanding*. The difference between chiropractic and other sciences and medical practices, however, is that most branches of medicine are much older and further removed from these roots on a mass scale despite still boldly showing their connections in the crests and emblems of every medical organization.

Chiropractic is still young, at roughly 125 years old, so these connections existed much closer to the present than other paradigms and have acted as a foundation that our practice was built on, not one we have actively tried to hide. That being said, and as mentioned above, most people do not even realize that the international symbol still used for medicine is the Caduceus staff, with the two serpent snakes of the Kundalini coiled around it. As far as the symbolism of the occult goes, they are rocking a pretty damn obvious one, but no one is the wiser.

In the following chapter, we will take a deeper look at some of the information that connects chiropractic to the esoteric understandings of the human body, as well as why the human body is believed to be the most sacred of all areas of study in ancient philosophy. Let's start with the above-mentioned Kundalini.

CHAPTER 6

THE KUNDALINI

The term Kundalini is of Sanskrit origin and translates loosely to "coiled serpent." It refers to a believed divine energy that is coiled and dormant at the base of the human spine, which, through meditation, intense practice, or Kundalini yoga training, can be drawn up the spinal cord to the crown of the head, which leads to an experience of rapid and dramatic enlightenment. Though this is something that can happen sometimes spontaneously, as reported by many people around the world, for most people, it is extremely difficult to achieve, even after spending a large portion of their lives training this skill. When the coiled serpent ascends all the way up the spine to its point of completion, it results in what is called a Kundalini awakening. The idea and practice of the Kundalini is intrinsically linked with the spine and depends on an unobstructed energetic flow up and down the spinal cord, from the coccyx to the base of the skull.

In this chapter, we are going to discuss the science behind Kundalini, its correlation to the science of chiropractic, and why the adjustment provides a potential benefit that quite literally no other treatment in the world can duplicate.

The idea of the Kundalini is a key to understanding the significance of the spinal cord and nervous system and why many cultures believe the power held within it holds the key to our divinity. Similarly, the chiropractic lens shares this view and recognizes the nervous system as the seat of human experience and is the primary focus in assessing and affecting all ailments and illnesses.

The Kundalini is spoken about as a single or pair of serpents that carry within them our divine wisdom. It is our inner connection to the source, our spiritual energy, and the potential path to our transcendence. In Kundalini practice, an individual learns to draw this winding serpent of energy up the spine by balancing the seven chakra points and conquering the impulses and desires of the lower self while learning to use these lessons as tools as they progress. The imagery here is quite significant, as serpent knowledge symbolism is shared through almost all ancient cultures and mythologies worldwide. Some examples of this known readily to Western cultures would be the serpent symbolism that is present in the Bible on multiple occasions, most notably in the creation myth of the Garden of Eden.

In the book of *Genesis*, the serpent tricked Eve into eating the fruit of the Tree of Knowledge. (Interestingly, gnostic Christians believe that the serpent in this situation was actually the benevolent God trying to free humanity from slavery under the jealous and lesser God of Yahweh – more on this theory is available in the books "The Gnostic Gospels," "Chariots of the Gods," and "The Gods of Eden.") The second major appearance of serpent symbolism in the Bible is in the book of *Numbers*, in which during the exodus from Egypt, when his people began to rebel and speak against Moses and his God Yahweh, this display of disrespect to God resulted in Yahweh sending out serpents to bite and kill the people who have betrayed him. In this story, after much pleading from the people to Moses for him to bargain with God, Moses is awarded a staff, which turns into a snake. He is told the staff would *save and protect all the people who gazed upon it.* This image calls to mind the picture of the modern Caduceus, which looks like a visual representation of the Kundalini. An image of this symbol can be seen on the front cover of Dr. Joe Dispenza's most recent book titled, "Becoming Supernatural."

Outside of Christian theology, the snake symbolism is even more prevalent in non-western parts of the world. In Mayan culture, the serpent was a very important social and religious symbol revered by the Mayans, along with the symbols of a powerful deity named Quetzalcoatl. Maya mythology describes serpents as being the vehicles by which celestial bodies, such as the sun and stars, cross the heavens. The shedding of their skin also made them a symbol of rebirth and renewal.

Snakes and Serpents are prevalent in the mythologies of the Hindu, Sumerian, Native American, and many other historical and modern cultures as well, usually representing some form of wisdom or knowledge from the divine.[3] For now, let's focus specifically on the snake symbolism in the form of the kundalini.

---

[3] This topic alone could fill an entire book, and if you are interested to learn more about these teachings and why they are relevant to the topic at hand, I suggest the book *The Secret Teachings of All Ages (1928)*, by Manly P. Hall.

The Kundalini energy is said to travel from the base of the sacrum up to the crown of the head, passing through the pineal gland en route to its final destination, resulting in the opening of the third eye. Along this path lie the seven Chakra points (some belief systems have nine or ten, which extend beneath the ground and up above the head in astral space). Though the number of chakra points and origins of the concept of wheels of energy that exist within our energetic anatomy spreads across many cultures with subtle variations, all versions of the Chakra systems share the same basic tenets. Let's take a look.

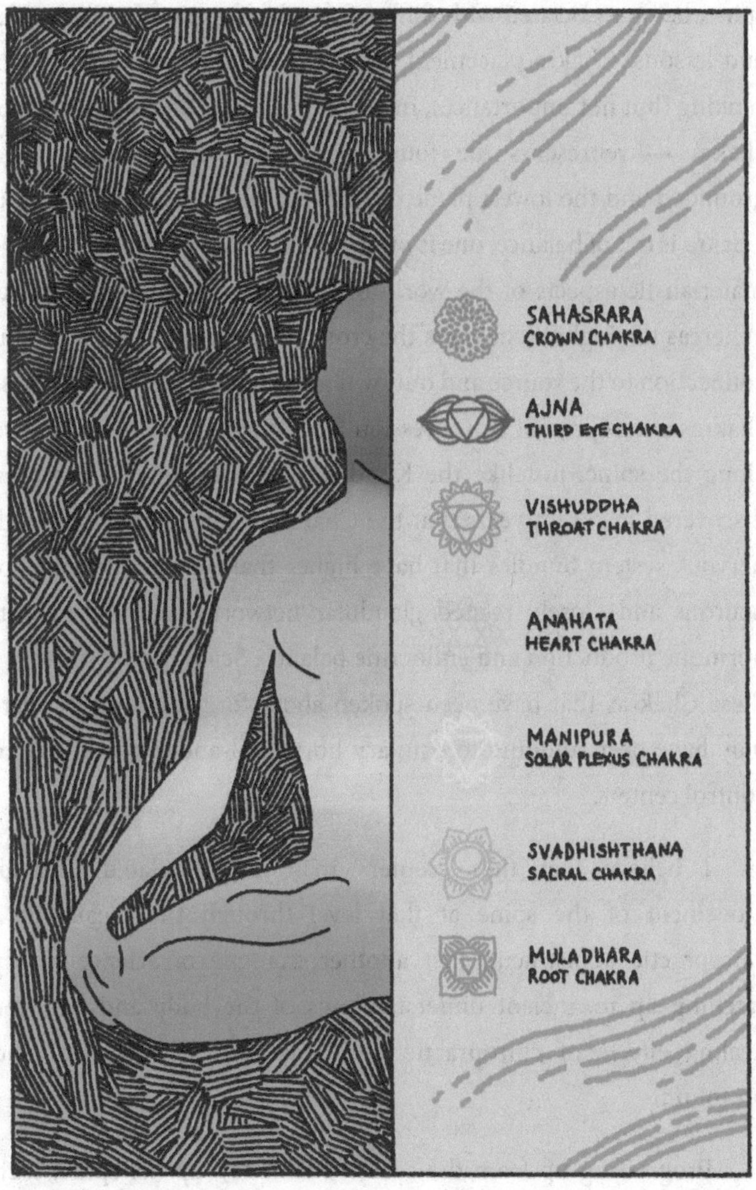

Each of the seven main Chakra points is shared across all systems, and each one corresponds to a different place along the spine, being associated with different levels of spiritual ability, gifts, and lessons. Chakra placement along the spine reflects an order of ranking (but not importance), in which the lowest chakra — the root chakra — represents the foundations of feeling connected or grounded and the lowest plane of spiritual development. When this Chakra is out of balance, one is often said to be bogged down with the materialistic aspects of the world or feelings of being ungrounded. Whereas the highest chakra is the crown Chakra and represents our connection to the source and our own true divinity. Notice how these chakras also represent a progression from material to divine upward along the spine, just like the Kundalini. Interestingly, it has been discovered in recent years that the Chakra centers correspond with nervous system bundles that have higher than normal densities of neurons and closely related glandular networks that control our hormone production and endocrine balance. Scientifically speaking, these Chakras that have been spoken about for thousands of years may have been alluding to primary hormonal and nervous system control centers.

I believe that these centers may be stimulated through movement of the spine at that level through the means of a chiropractic adjustment. Just another example of science slowly catching up to ancient understandings of the body and why the healing effects of chiropractic care may be so widespread and profound.

Progressing up from the coccyx (tailbone), up the spine, each section of the vertebra is closely linked with a specific chakra, or as mentioned, a specific branch of our endocrine and nervous systems. Let's look at the root and sacral Chakras, for example:

Directly running in front of the sacrum is what is called the sacral plexus. It's a hub of sympathetic ganglions (large bulbs of dense nerve fibers) that regulate and control the sympathetic and parasympathetic nervous system balance in the lower extremities. In English, for my non-nerd folk, this controls the fight or flight mechanism in your legs, which regulates blood flow, muscle tension, and sensation in the lower limbs. When your blood vessels are constricted in your legs, creating altered or strange sensations due to overstimulation of the sympathetic nervous system from a sacrum distortion, this can lead to an altered experience of your lower limb sensation. This makes your muscles extra tight and constricts your lower limb blood vessels, limiting oxygen, as your ability to interpret sensation from the ground becomes diminished. The scientific explanation is a natural and well-understood result of a sacrum distortion, but the lived experience, the experience within the individuals with this pattern, can lead to numb and cold feet, or restless leg syndrome. Both result in quite literally a sensation of being ungrounded and disconnected from the physical earth and your lower body. So again, we see that the science may line up with the ancient understanding, only we are still so far behind in our wisdom in the Western world that we haven't quite connected the dots yet.

For another example, we can also look at the thoracic spine (behind the shoulder blades), in which we have a chain of nerve bundles called the sympathetic trunk that runs down both sides of the thoracic vertebrae all the way from our first thoracic vertebra down to our 11th. If you look at the image below, you will see how it divides up into different sections that control different internal organs. I would like you to note the cardiac plexus, which is associated with the heart Chakra, and also note the anterior vagal trunk — the extremity of the very much talked about vagus nerve,[4] which correlates with the Solar plexus Chakra. Look at the two images below and compare areas of nervous system bundles with the Chakra points. You can see that perhaps these ancient Vedic and chakra-based traditions were onto something much more profound than just the simple New Age understanding.

---

[4] More on this in the books "Activating the Healing Power of the Vagus Nerve" by Stanley Rosenberg, or "The Polyvagal Theory" by Stephen W. Porges.

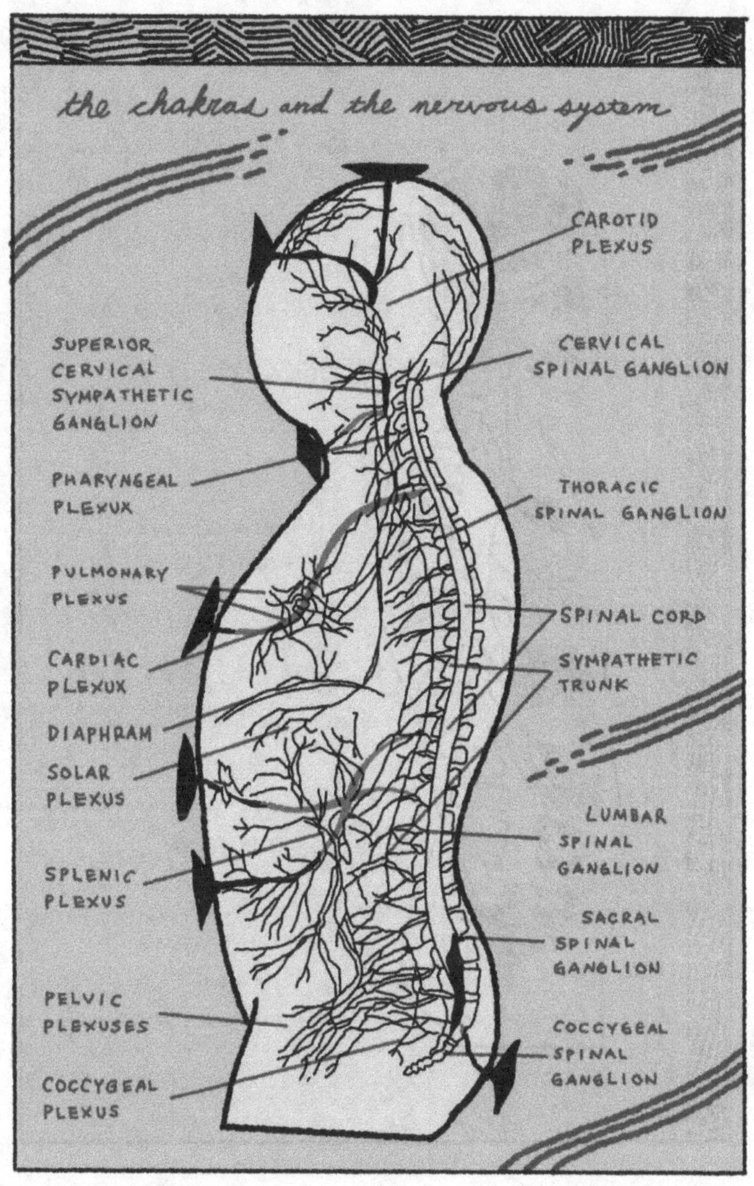

the chakras and the nervous system
CAROTID PLEXUS
SUPERIOR CERVICAL SYMPATHETIC GANGLION
CERVICAL SPINAL GANGLION
PHARYNGEAL PLEXUX
THORACIC SPINAL GANGLION
PULMONARY PLEXUS
CARDIAC PLEXUX
SPINAL CORD
SYMPATHETIC TRUNK
DIAPHRAM
SOLAR PLEXUS
LUMBAR SPINAL GANGLION
SPLENIC PLEXUS
SACRAL SPINAL GANGLION
PELVIC PLEXUSES
COCCYGEAL SPINAL GANGLION
COCCYGEAL PLEXUS

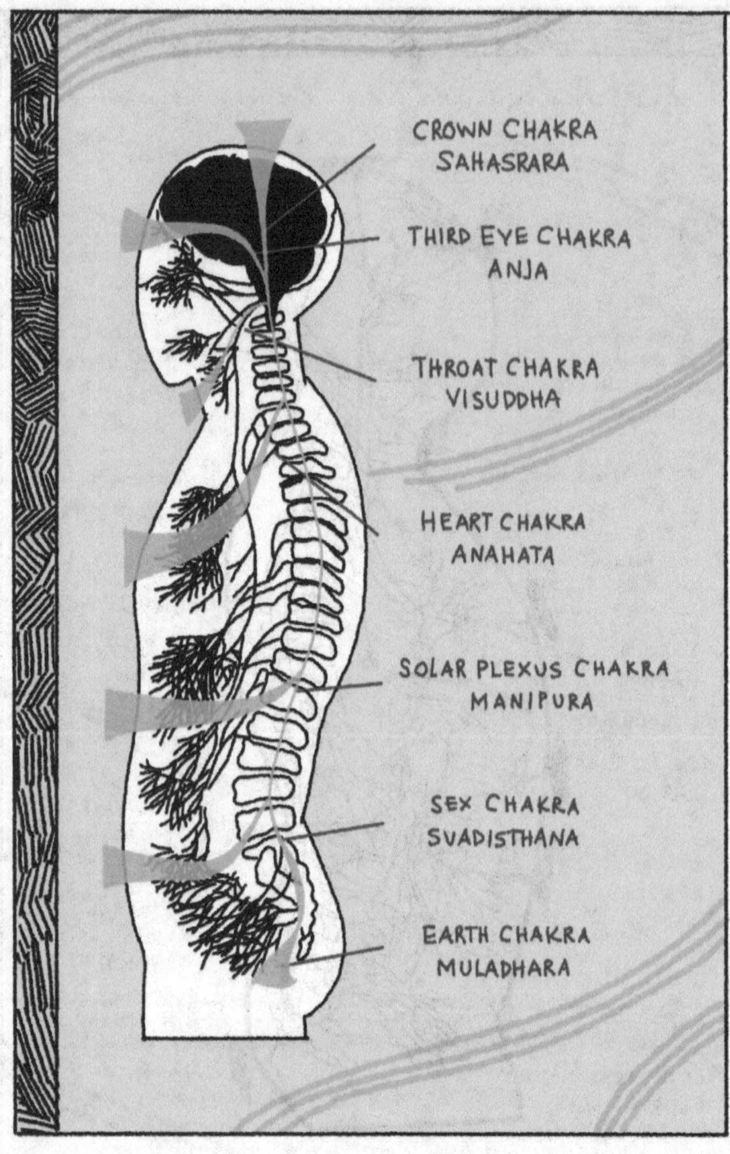

So if we can trace out these points and show their anatomical connection with specific areas of the spine, and we can demonstrate scientifically what a distortion at that area of the spine would result in symptomatically, and show that same pattern correlates with the wisdom of what an imbalance at that specific chakra would present as, then how can we use this combined knowledge to hack our health and maximize our overall expression?

A chiropractic adjustment is a very specific and fast motion given to a very specific vertebra in a very specific direction to restore proper alignment and neurological function to that area along with its affected anatomy. An adjustment can also be used to stimulate these nerve and endocrine centers, forcing the brain to check in on each one of these areas at a higher rate than it would if no adjustment was provided.

According to research done at the Haavik Research Centre in New Zealand by the chiropractor and neurophysiologist Dr. Heidi Haavik, it has been shown that a chiropractic adjustment stimulates the nerve bundles around the vertebral segment being adjusted, as well as the Golgi tendon fibers in the muscles surrounding that segment (cells designed to respond to stretch in the muscle), resulting in the stimulation of the prefrontal cortex of the brain as it interprets and responds to these signals. The prefrontal cortex is the central control center of the brain and the hub of executive decision-making inside the nervous system.

Aka you.

To simplify, the adjustment instantly affects the main control and interpretation center of the brain, along with the local area and neurology of the segment being adjusted. Even simpler: every adjustment affects and changes both the body and the brain.

So, what if you provide an adjustment to an area of the spine that is associated with a chakra center? Well, in my opinion, you would be systematically stimulating the chakra center, along with the nerve and endocrine centers associated with it and facilitating a connection and communication between these centers and the main control center of the brain. If done often enough, this could create a higher level of recalibration to these chakra balances than any other form of treatment, which could help expedite and support internal efforts and training to achieve a kundalini awakening or to simply balance your energetic centers. If a full awakening is not something you care to achieve, at the very least, I believe that these consistent recalibrations would result in higher levels of overall hormonal and nervous system balance in the body, inevitably resulting in a healthier, more balanced human experience.

Now, something important to note about the research done by Haavik is that it was stated that one of the most fundamental parts of the adjustment that is required to create this response is the *speed* at which it is delivered.

The adjustments performed by a skilled chiropractor are unlike any other manipulations done in other professions. Though many other branches of medicine and manual therapy have attempted to borrow and adopt manipulation (they call them manipulations, chiropractors prefer to call them adjustments) into their services, none of them come close to the same level of training and precision in applying this skill as a trained and experienced chiropractor.

An adjustment, as performed by most chiropractic techniques, is a high velocity, low amplitude movement, meaning a fast but small movement in the direction a joint is designed to go. It is performed with greater speed and directed precision than that of the high velocity, low amplitude (HVLA) movements of manual therapy, physiotherapy, massage, and osteopathy. Interestingly, according to Haavik, speed is actually a large requirement for the stimulation of the prefrontal cortex in the desired way she shows in her research.

Now, I would like to make a caveat here that there are also gentle techniques of chiropractic that are extremely effective at clearing the pathway in the upper cervical area, which can lead to profound healing as well, and the manipulations mentioned above as performed by other practicing modalities can also be valid and effective as well at providing great results; however, for the specific topic we are addressing, only high-speed, specific adjustments can stimulate the nervous system in the way required to have the effects shown in Haavik's work.[5]

Circling back to the initial topic of the Kundalini, why would a high-speed, specific chiropractic adjustment be helpful in the ascension of the Kundalini energy up the spinal column? Well, you see, in some ways, the chiropractic profession may have stumbled across a way to hack the Kundalini by quite simply cracking the Kundalini.

---

[5] For more on Dr. Haavik and her team, you can find her book "The Reality Check," as well as her published and peer reviewed studies at: https://therealitycheck.com.

CLEARING THE ROADBLOCKS

Firstly, as a chiropractor, when looking at the spine, we look for areas that have the highest amount of stress due to fixation or dysfunction. This stress can be shown as an increased tone in the muscle around the joint, increased resistance to movement in the articulations, swelling, heat, and limited or paradoxical movement. In his paradigm shifting book, *The Body Electric* (1985), Robert O. Becker explains how stress causes the tissues in the muscle and bone to change their electrical signature. This electrical change can not only lead to inflammation but also inhibit the nerves in the area from sending and receiving signals at their highest capacity and optimal speed. Remember, nerves are electric in nature, so when you change the current around a nerve, you change the function of the nerve. This becomes quite literally an *electrical* roadblock for the Kundalini to have to travel past, and one that can affect the function of both the local tissues as well as the tissues and organs with which that nerve communicates.

Secondly, the discs and spinal cord in that area are nourished by fluids that are circulated around them at all times and are stimulated by the movement of the spine in a process called imbibition. Imbibition is when the proper movement of each spinal segment is used to pump fluid up and down the spinal cord and nourish that vertebral disc, surrounding tissues, and each level of the spinal cord. Spinal segments that do not move do not create imbibition, so there will be a pooling of cellular waste in the fluids of that area and a lack of fresh nutrients reaching that segment, which leads to a *chemical* roadblock for the Kundalini current and a blind spot in the bodies surveillance system. Over 70% of all stimulation the brain gets each day comes from these movements of spinal segments. Each movement is a signal the brain uses to understand the body's internal and external environment at each level and collectively as a whole. When there is a lack of natural movement, there is not only a lack of imbibition, but there is a disruption to the body's communication and ability to interpret the world it is in, both its internal world as well as its external world.

Thirdly, when these areas have been under stress for a long enough period, bone will follow the signals of the changed electrical current and begin to grow in the form of degenerative joint disease and as a last-ditch effort to stabilize the area over time.

Finally, if there is an acute injury to the area and either the vertebra is displaced, or a disc becomes herniated, then these conditions represent possible *physical* and *mechanical* roadblocks to the Kundalini, in which a physical compression of a nerve can more severally limit the communication and function of that nerve and its affected limb or organ. As a chiropractor, we seek the various signs of these roadblocks, and within our profession, the combination of an electrical, chemical, and mechanical roadblock is summed up in the term *Subluxation*, which translates literally to "less light". These subluxations lead to lower levels of health and function in each area, and cumulatively each one of these disruptions adds to and amplifies the next by further distorting the communication signals. If one security camera goes out, you have a blind spot and potential risk; if three, four, five, or more cameras go out, then you have a completely ineffective surveillance system.

As chiropractors, we find and adjust subluxations, thus removing the trifold roadblocks and clearing the pathways for the kundalini by re-establishing proper imbibition, chemical, electrical, and physical balance in the area and to the organs in which that area communicates. Without further interference, the body can heal itself. This is our philosophy.

This connection to ancient philosophies of spiritual ascension through proper energetic transmission up and down the spinal cord is one of the most profound yet neglected sides of collective current scientific study. Even within the chiropractic profession, we have spent so much time trying to demonstrate the effects of an adjustment on pain, which I am all for in that there have been some groundbreaking studies on the benefits of chiropractic for pain management and the prevention of opioid use; however, I believe we have turned our attention too completely into the pain side of what we do that we have ignored the more profound effects of chiropractic.

The basis of chiropractic philosophy, art, and science was founded on a mixture of scientific and esoteric understandings of the human body. These understandings were vastly ahead of their time, which unfortunately led to scrutiny and opposition by the existing and dominant allopathic model. However, as we have begun to demonstrate, current science is always playing catch up, and I believe a more vitalistic approach to health and healing is an idea whose time has finally come.

Chiropractic is only about 130 years old, and It's usually not until many years after a new or newly remembered idea hits the public that scientific understanding eventually begins to catch up. At this point, we tend to see a sudden acceptance of previously ridiculed ideas as recognized and obvious facts, just like the sun revolving around the earth. I believe we are reaching that turning point for not only chiropractic but all other natural healing modalities that have taken their understanding from old teachings and applied them appropriately and effectively. The empirical world has a nasty habit of taking ideas from the spiritual teachings of ancient cultures years after they were originally introduced and likely burned to the ground, studying them in secret, then disregarding their origin and claiming them as their own inventions. As seemingly unbelievable as this may be, this same pattern is just as pervasive and just as true in medicine as it is in any other scientific pursuit. Perhaps even more so.

Remember the Caduceus that we mentioned earlier being the international symbol of medicine used to this day? This symbol, which was taken from Hermes Trismegistus of ancient Greece (who was said to be a reincarnation of Thoth from ancient Egypt and the God of wisdom), demonstrates the dual Kundalini serpent climbing up the spinal cord to the crown of the head in the process described above. So, the international symbol of medicine represents the Kundalini energy of spiritual ascension given to us by the reincarnation of the God of wisdom. Does that make *any* sense to you unless there was some hidden previous occult connection? I feel this would be a much more fitting symbol for chiropractic than medicine.

Side note: While at an appointment for my dad with an eye specialist, I looked at the certificates on the wall of the specialist he was seeing. To my utter surprise and amusement, the symbol used for the seal of the Medical Council of Canada has a dragon on one side, a unicorn on the other, and two serpents at the top eating their own tails — another famous occult image called the ouroboros. Can you explain that one to me if they are not hinting at esoteric connections?

Because I sure as shit can't.

—⟶∞⟵—

CHAPTER 7

THE BODY AS A BATTERY

It is a well-established fact that the human body is an electric entity. Albeit a complicated one, but nonetheless, it is essentially a battery. Electricity is the medium in which we send and receive signals to and from the brain carrying information, as discussed in the previous chapter. It is also the driving energy behind the sensations associated with the ascent of the Kundalini and why a stronger current of electricity can result in a stronger and more robust life force inside the body. The simple act of being alive for any tissue in the body is based on the properties of electricity running through it and animating it. We are the same as a cell phone: no electric charge, no life.

Let's think about electricity a little bit deeper and break it down in relation to our diet.

When it comes to our diets, we all seem to think of nutrition as a discussion focused on macronutrients (fats vs. proteins vs. carbohydrates), and we endlessly obsess over calories in versus calories out for goals like fat loss or muscle gain and simple macronutrient ratios. Adding to the confusion of this debate are the ideas of the various concepts such as If It Fits Your Macros (IIFYM), Carnivore vs. Vegan, Keto, Carb loading, ethical eating, plant-based, and on and on. When you try and sift through it all, you are usually left feeling defeated and hopeless.

The online nutrition world, just like the fitness world discussed in the introduction, is filled with influencers yelling their secret miracle diets at the masses while making shit piles of money as helpless and desperate people bounce from one idea to another while throwing their money at whatever comes their way, hoping to find the hidden gem that has eluded them their entire lives. These nutritional concepts sell an illusion of health, all while missing the single most important fact about food: the food you eat, including macro *and* micronutrients, dictate the *quality and level of electrical conductance within your body and supply the building blocks available to form your tissues.*

When it comes to human cellular health, the higher the conductance, the healthier the individual and the less their system has to work to use energy (calories) effectively to function, and the higher the quality of resources available to form building blocks, the more accurately the body can follow the energetic blueprint to build your tissues. The more electricity and the greater the conductance, the stronger the blueprint; the higher the quality of building blocks, the more accurately your body can build a quality structure using those blueprints.

In contrast, a less healthy individual has lower energy to begin with, and coupled with an insulated body that is resistant to conduction and poorer quality materials for building blocks, this individual's body needs to work significantly harder to distribute electricity to all of its cells, while trying to follow a less clear blueprint and using lower quality materials for building blocks.

You can imagine two home builders: one who has a clear and concise plan drawn up by an architect with attention to detail, and a contractor who settles for no less than the absolute best quality work and materials; and the second, who has a basic blueprint but a contractor who cuts corners and is always looking for a bargain on materials. You can imagine which house will turn out better. Even if the second one looks beautiful when it is finished, will the quality of the build stand the test of time?

Many people aren't aware of this, but the heart is the prime electrical source of our bodies, not our brains. Does it make more sense that heart disease is so prevalent among overweight individuals now? The heart has to work extra hard to distribute electricity to all areas of the body because the sheer size of the body itself has become less efficient, and the makeup of the body's tissues is out of balance, resulting in reduced electrical transmission.

The things that affect electrical transmission most are body fat content, mineral and electrolyte balance, and toxin exposure. Let me show you.

IT'S THE LITTLE THINGS THAT KILL... OR HEAL

When you are boiling a pot of water and want it to hurry up, what do you do?

You put salt in the water.

Why?

Because salt increases the energy conductance rate in the water, causing the pot to boil faster. Salt has electrons in it, acting as electrolytes in the water, allowing the water to carry and pass an electrical current faster. Now, if you notice, our saliva is also somewhat salty for the same reason, and so is our sweat. All our bodily fluids have a level of saltiness within them because they are all not only water-based but are also organic fluids, which means they are electrically charged.

Our bodies are an intricate balance of salts, minerals, and micronutrients that are fundamentally important for our cells to work on a micro level and greatly influence how our bodies work on a macro level. The sodium-potassium balance is one of the most important ratios in our bodies, yet I highly doubt any diet you have ever tried spoke about it. In fact, I would also wager that no doctor you have ever seen has mentioned it either — other than potentially villainizing salt and telling you to eat less of it along with red meat and eggs.

We are being taught that salt is bad and we should limit salt intake for things like heart disease prevention and high blood pressure; however, the actual truth is that an *elevated salt-to-potassium ratio* is what is bad, not salt itself.

In fact, salt is essential.

This ratio is one of the basic balances that helps to maintain appropriate electrical conductance in our bodies and, thus, cellular function and health. As with most things in life, with every organism and every process within that organism, there is a sweet spot. The effort to stay in this sweet spot is called homeostasis, and it is what your body strives for at all times, in all ways. You need all the ingredients, but just like baking a cookie, you need them all within a certain range and at certain ratios to function optimally. If your cookies have a little more salt in them or a little less sugar, they will still taste fairly good. That is until you pass a certain limit. Put way too much or way too little of any one of those ingredients, and you end up with shit cookies. Fact.

If you start to look at food and drinks on a micronutrient level instead of a surface macro level, you will begin to see a completely different world of nutrition and may have a few lightbulb moments in the grocery store aisle.

I want to take an aside to address one of the ideas mentioned in a few paragraphs above that I believe is detrimental to long-term health when you understand the electrical importance of food.

I will say it now and hope not to offend anyone, but the fad concept of "If It Fits Your Macros," (IIFYS) is single-handedly the dumbest nutritional concept in existence on a micronutrient level.

I'm sorry, but someone had to say it.

At its onset, it was designed as a simple way to count calories and achieve an aesthetic goal without overcomplicating dieting. It works fine for that goal because most bodybuilding and competitive aesthetic techniques are far from health-oriented anyway, and the people competing are fully aware of it. As long as you are using IIFYM with that basic understanding, then the concept isn't so bad, and power to you. The problem comes when the concept of IIFYM is taken too far out of context and placed into long-term usage for the masses. All of a sudden, an easy short-term dieting hack becomes a long-term health risk.

Due to its short-term goal success and simplicity, we now have non-competitive athletes using IIFYM as a blueprint for their long-term health and weight directives, not knowing that it was never intended for this application. This is a massive problem because it is an incredibly dangerous oversimplification of nutrition, which leads to an obscured concept of food value for the individuals using it. Logically, when you think about it, the very concept itself is ludicrous to promote when you understand any basic nutrition, but it is trendy and gets results, so it caught on like fire. Just in case you have never heard of it, let me explain IIFYM to you.

The basic idea of IIFYM is that as long as a food is within the same macronutrient category as another food (fats, carbs, or proteins), then an equal number of calories of that food is exactly equal in the body to the same number of calories of the other food. A clean and easy exchange. One carb for another carb. Simple.

This is the allure; you can have fifty calories of a donut instead of fifty calories of a potato or boring old rice. No biggie, your body is really dumb, and you can pull a fast one on it. It can't even tell the difference! Right?!

I'm sorry, but no.

Fifty calories of a donut are not equal to fifty calories of rice, which are also not equal to fifty calories of potato or fifty calories of any other carbohydrate you can name. Just because they are all fifty calories of a food considered to be a carbohydrate does not in any way mean that they have the same nutritional value to the body and have the exact same effect on your health. Not a chance.

Every single piece of food has both its *macro* calorie components and, more importantly, its *unique chemical composition that encompasses its micronutrient components*. When understood on this level, fifty calories of a donut aren't even comparable to fifty calories of a different brand or flavor of donut, let alone fifty calories of any other type of food, carbohydrate or not! We have to start using these squishy things inside of skulls when evaluating information in the health and fitness industries, regardless if it comes from the mainstream, an influencer, or an "expert."

FATS: THEIR TRUE PURPOSE IN OUR BODIES

Let's talk about what's inside the elephant in the room.

Adipose tissue, aka *fat*.

I might as well start with the boldest statement right off the bat: *Everything you know about fat is wrong.* At the very least, it is wholly incomplete.

Fat in the body does not build up because you ate too much fat.

Taking fat in does not equal fat stored. We can thank the sugar and cereal industries for the propaganda that told us it did, as they successfully deflected the attention from themselves for the problems they were creating by blaming it on a macronutrient that didn't really have any large corporations backing it.

So I will repeat this again: fat does not build up because you ate too many calories of fat and it needs somewhere to store them because you haven't burned them off. Fat doesn't even build up because you love cake and can't put down the chocolate and red wine. Fat has one main lifesaving job outside of the small amounts of insulation it provides: Fat walls off toxins in the body when the liver cannot process them fast enough.

Read that again.

Fat is a life-saving substance that takes toxins within your body from the shitty quality food you eat, the polluted and recycled air you breathe in, or the alcohol you drink, and it walls them off when your liver cannot process and detox them fast enough. Your body can only process a certain amount of toxins at a time, so this is where the surplus in calories has an effect in that if the body has too many toxins carried within those calories, but more are coming in before it can process the ones already existing, it will use fat to wall them off to deal with them later when there is a deficit in calorie and toxin intake.

The healthier you are, and the more efficient your organ's function, the better it can detox harmful chemicals from the body. However, if you are constantly adding harmful chemicals and toxins to your body at a higher rate than it can process, then your body cannot keep up and will begin the process of fat storage to package up those toxins in the idea that if they can't be processed now, then putting them in a container and storing them to process later is a better option than allowing your body to be subject to a toxin overload. This is the reason why some people seem to store fat like it's an Olympic sport, and others can eat a stick of butter every hour and continue to look like bones and sinew. This is also why extremely fast weight loss is genuinely unhealthy and sometimes potentially dangerous because you are quickly freeing all these toxins from your storage units, and the body is being bombarded with those toxins as it struggles to process and excrete them.

The good news is your body is insanely good at not dying, so even though it is not healthy, it can usually do a pretty good job of processing those toxins as long as very low levels of new toxins are coming in, so as not to tax its resources and overwork your liver. This fact alone is why literally all diets that involve eating healthier food with less toxins and lower calories work, regardless of whether that food is plant, juice, or animal based.

Did veganism save your life? Are you a die-hard keto enthusiast because it cured you of Type-2 diabetes? Are you on the juicing train because you are dropping weight like the dollar bills you spend on fresh organic veggies? Well, spoiler alert, you are getting results mostly because you actually just started eating healthy food and cut out all the shit. It's amazing how good you can feel when you eat *real* food exclusively and stop filling yourself with toxic chemicals and man-made synthetic foods.

Now that we understand fat's main purpose, let's get back to the electrical properties of the body and why fat has an important effect on them and can have such a big impact on your overall health.

Fat is like rubber. It's an insulator, meaning electricity does not readily flow through it, and neither does water. This is why it is so effective at walling off and storing toxins. So, when we previously discussed how it is important to balance micronutrient and mineral intake to maximize electrical efficiency, well, fat is pretty much the exact opposite of that desired efficiency and the biggest conductance reducer in the body. Not only does fat wall off all your toxins, but it also stops electrical energy from traveling through your body at its most efficient rate. Therefore, if you gave 100 calories to an individual with low body fat and 100 calories to an individual with high body fat, you would see that the individual with low body fat would use those calories more efficiently throughout the body because less energy is needed to pass them from one tissue to the next, so less energy is lost as it travels.

Now, with all things human, the simplicity of this is only presented as a teaching tool because, as any athlete out there with a large portion of muscle mass who is reading this is probably ready to scream at me knows, more muscle mass equals more calories needed to operate as well. Despite an individual being electrically efficient, they still may require high levels of calories to function optimally because they have more high-performing tissue requirements, so their body uses more electrical energy to fuel performance instead of lost electrical energy due to inefficiency— think a Ferrari engine versus a Hyundai engine. I'm quite sure that the Ferrari engineers are better at creating efficiency and power than the Hyundai engineers; however, your Ferrari may require premium fuel and a lot more of it to go the same distance. If you create a high-performance engine, it requires better fuel and more of it.

On the opposite side of things, an individual who has a high body-fat ratio and much less muscle mass may also require a ton of calories in a day — but they require them for a different reason. They are a Hyundai towing a trailer. More energy is required due to lost efficiency.

When the body is heavily insulated both inside and out, then a single calorie doesn't go nearly as far because its energy is wasted trying to pass through impassable barriers. Multiple calories may be needed to perform the same tasks. Think about the difference like this: a heavily muscled individual, while on a hiking trip, may be carrying 220 pounds of total weight, but they *are* that weight, and each muscle is part of the function of that weight. In contrast, an individual that is 220 pounds of body weight but has a high fat ratio functions more like an individual who weighs 170 pounds hiking while carrying a 50-pound backpack. The weight of those fat cells does not contribute to the overall function of the individual and becomes extra weight. Thus, both people require similar calories to make it up the mountain, but for drastically different reasons.

To complete the picture, the individual that is 170 lbs. with a low-fat ratio is going to require lower calories than both because they have higher efficiency as well less excess weight, useful or not. I would also like to mention that there is a bottom limit to healthy body fat. Remembering that the body is an electrical unit, we must remember that all of our internal organs are highly electrical as well and need to function independently, so some purposeful electrical barriers are necessary.

We have two kinds of fat: subcutaneous fat, which is the fat that lies under our skin, and epithelial tissues. Visceral fat is the fat that surrounds our organs inside of our abdomen. Despite high levels of visceral fat being the more dangerous of the two, some levels of visceral fat are needed to maintain healthy organ function for exactly the reason we have just stated above: insulation. Too much insulation is bad, but some insulation is necessary. It's another example of a sweet spot our body always strives for.

Think about the necessary visceral fat like this: when you are wiring the electrical in a house, the wires are surrounded by a plastic coating to make sure they do not touch each other accidentally and cause cross-firing, or electrical damage. The same principles govern our organs. Without some level of fat to insulate them and separate them from each other, they would be just like multiple live wires butted up against each other inside us. In this circumstance, insulation is needed to allow proper function, but only a small amount. This is why having lowered levels of fat in the body can be problematic as well, but only a small fraction of people would ever have to worry about passing this limit. It is very difficult to obtain and not something that most people have to worry about unless you intend to be stage-ready for a bodybuilding contest 365 days a year.

Another reason fat levels are dangerous if they drop too low — and why it is dangerous to eliminate fat from our diet completely— is that fat and cholesterol are required for cell membrane maintenance and neuron function in the brain. Neurons (brain cells) inside the brain come in two distinct categories: myelinated and unmyelinated. The myelinated form comes with a myelin sheath wrapped around the neuron that allows for insulation and faster nerve impulse transmission. The building blocks used to form myelin are derived from fats in the body. These myelin sheaths are integral to maintaining proper neurological and physical function. When these sheaths begin to degrade, an individual experiences one of the many types of Demyelinating diseases; the most readily recognized is one called Multiple Sclerosis.

On top of these very important structures, other equally important structures require fat in the form of cholesterol to function, such as the membrane of every single cell in your body. This means that low-cholesterol diets and medication that reduces cholesterol production may actually be putting us at risk of damage to these membranes and myelin sheaths.

The purpose of this chapter was to draw attention to the effects of nutrition on the electrical functions of the body, how fat can affect the electrical efficiency of the body, and why these electrical effects matter to your overall health. The body is, at its core, when speaking energetically, a complicated battery. How this living battery charges and depletes itself is quite varied and diverse. Many of these avenues of energy gain or energy loss may be logical to you, such as through the consumption of energy in the base of food, but some may have been less obvious, such as the electrical properties of minerals and micronutrients and the importance of body composition as detailed above.

As we progress through to the final chapter of this book, we will take a look at less obvious and likely surprising topics that relate to managing and optimizing our own internal energy stores, but first, let's take a look at some of the other important rules and processes of the body that may, or may not be new ways of thinking that will begin to reshape and remold your ideas about this awe-inspiring soul vehicle that we live in.

We will begin to shift from the material, physical processes and rules of the body into the more subtle but profound realms of conscious control and effect on our physical, emotional, and energetic realities. We'll also look at the importance of understanding our true nature as divine beings existing simultaneously as the bodies in which we experience the world through our five senses, but also somehow much more beyond that. Our true essence inhabits our bodies but is also above our bodies. As we go forward, our essence is something I will be referring to as *episomatic*.

Epi= Above, Somatic= Our Body

CHAPTER 8

OUR EPISOMATIC NATURE

When we genuinely place our intention on understanding our true nature, not just our superficial and physical nature, most individuals eventually come to the realization that we are both simultaneously our bodies and not our bodies at the same time.

Historical mystical texts, as well as modern metaphysical and new age ideas borrowed from traditional philosophies, show a consistent understanding that we are divine beings that exist in essence outside of our bodies and, therefore, are not synonymous with our bodies. Still, our bodies, in this reality we experience every day, are incredibly real and should not be discounted. We are individual emanations of divine energy experiencing a unique moment, and each unto ourselves is a divine being that exists in a form that has, and will, transcend our bodies to exist eternally in some form or another.

Despite this, we also come across the undeniable truth that regardless of these divine and everlasting properties of ourselves, we are currently bound to our physical bodies to experience life through their five senses and bound in this material world by its laws. No matter how much we try to ignore either of these aspects, we cannot escape them.

Combining these two distinct but equally true aspects of ourselves in our current experience and expression of life, we are, as both divine and human beings, something I have called *Episomatic*. This term translates literally to "above the body," and represents the understanding of this dual existence we are currently in.

I have created this term to use here because I believe the term *episomatic* more accurately describes *what we are* than any other term I have been able to come across; therefore, I felt it necessary to place a new distinction and definition on the idea. This term encompasses not only the idea that we are divine and infinite entities that exist outside of and independent of our bodies but also the understanding that despite this, while we are present in human form, we are physical expressions of that divine blueprint in an earth-bound form as well. We are simultaneously our bodies, but not our bodies. Our bodies are a single-dimensional aspect of our divine selves, which ultimately exists beyond our bodies.

THE PHYSICAL BODY

Despite some branches of spiritual thought, such as the Gnostics, believing that our bodies are prisons and that we must work tirelessly to gain the wisdom to free ourselves from, or many New Age authors pushing the idea that we are not our bodies at all and therefore should not pay attention to, or identify with them; I do not hold these views and believe it is necessary to create a distinction between them and the Episomatic reality I have presented here. I believe that our bodies are us, and I believe our bodies are the greatest gift that has ever been bestowed on us because it is through the use of and experience of our bodies that we are able to experience and interact with every other aspect and experience of existence that we have had as humans; which for most of us, that is all we have ever known or remember.

To disregard our bodies and attempt to demonize them is to demonize the greatest gift we have ever received. Perhaps, as divine spirits, when we all ascend to our next form of existence, we will feel some relief as we shed these restricting confines — much like a snake does its skin. However, while we exist here on this earth and in this lifetime, we do not have the option of existing without our bodies and shedding this current form, nor do I think we would want to. It is part of our duty and life purpose to use and master these bodies, to help us create and experience any and everything we desire and long for in this form while cultivating a moral distinction as we weigh and experience the outcomes of our decisions.

Think about the importance of truly identifying with and feeling grateful for your body and all the experiences it has to offer. Have you ever watched a sunset so beautiful that everything else in your life slowed down and vanished for those few moments? Your eyes granted you that experience. Have you ever felt the soft, warm lips of a loved one as they kissed you when you needed it most? Your lips, skin, and physical form are the only reason you were able to experience that. Or the smell of cherry blossoms in the springtime. Our bodies are the greatest treasures we have, and it is our job to honor them while also honoring and acknowledging our divine essence. As many people have said many times before, our bodies are temples. We must learn how they work and respect them at all costs.

THE COMPLEXITY OF OUR MATERIAL BODIES

Our bodies *are us* as we know them to be, but they are also composed of diverse and countless material building blocks that make them intricately connected to and part of this vast world of material reality in which we live. Despite our bodies being our personal vehicles and avatars through which we live, experience, and interact with the material world, our bodies also contain atoms, electrons, and subatomic particles that have existed before us as trees, plants, jaguars, wolves, whales, humans, stars, planets, and potentially all other variations of material things that existed in our world, and universe, at some point in time.

We have trillions of cells in our bodies, which are made up of countless trillions of atoms and particles. You likely have within you atoms from every other form of existence in the universe at one time or another. This is possible because, despite being unique individuations of physical entities, we all share the same base building blocks of structure that are constantly recycling and exchanging with the physical world. Our bodies, therefore, and the physical forms of every other person, animal, and all other physical things in existence energetically and materially consist of tiny pieces that have been shared and actively exchanged back and forth on a daily basis since the beginning of time. This is the scientific proof that we are all connected, and we are all part of the same vast, all-encompassing oneness.

Even the simple act of breathing is one way in which we take part in this exchange every second of our lives. We breathe in oxygen, nitrogen, carbon monoxide, and dioxide, among other gaseous components that have existed inside and sometimes as part of other people's bodies before being taken up into our own. They carry subtle signatures of all of the previous forms of existence they have contributed to and are converted into various elements that our body uses to create tissue and perform cellular functions. Once this internal integration process is complete inside our lungs, these atoms and particles shift and change — sometimes back into similar forms, sometimes into different ones — to complete the cycle by being expelled back out into the world and made available to be taken up by other individuals. What this means is that with every single breath you take, your body is taking in and absorbing information and elements that have come from countless other things and beings before you and breathing back out into the world information from you and units of matter to be used by someone or something else in an infinite and beautiful information exchange.

Other forms of this energetic, physical, and information exchange come through the processes of consumption of food and water, as well as the absorption of chemicals and energy through the skin. Your body, in fact, has never been a constant and isolated thing but instead has been an active participant in a divine symphony of events and processes using temporary actors and agents to exist in the physical realm. This symphony combines forces and building blocks of the material and electromagnetic world with the divine will of consciousness that is the guiding, cohesive force responsible for making up and maintaining us as physical things in this physical reality.

What this means is that despite the common understanding many of us have about the collective consciousness in which we all are part of and connected through our shared subconscious — much like individual waves in the vastness of the ocean — we are also connected just as intimately in the physical plane. I hope that this can provide you with a new appreciation of your physical body and give you a profound feeling of trust in the wisdom within them. Our bodies, after all, hold the wisdom of the entirety of creation.

THE DIVINE SELF

While we have a physical structure, which allows us to exist as part of the material world, it is also true that we are not *just* our bodies; rather, we are something even more profound. More all-encompassing. More inspiring.

Our true selves and essence exist within the divine spark of our souls. Our essence, in truth, is incomprehensible, but we can think of it as the pure light that radiates into our bodies from the divine realm, being distilled and dispersed into all corners of our physical frames. This pure light is what animates us. It lends its energy and understanding to our sensory organs, interpreting their messages and formulating them into experiences of the material world while eternally connecting us to the All of existence.

Without this light projected into our tissues, and without the divine essence of what and who we are being transmitted into our physical bodies at all times, our bodies and tissues would instantaneously begin to decay, kick-starting the process of entropy by regressing into the elementary and base particles of which they consist, and returning them to the pool of possibility that is used to constantly create the material world. When divine light leaves our body, our bodies no longer are us but a collection of physical building blocks that will degrade and be used again to create something else.

Our divine light, our divine selves, and our pure essence are the energetic, magnetic, and conscious force that holds us together in *order* and fights against the powerful natural force of decay called entropy. Entropy is the scientific principle in which all objects and beings in the material world move towards decay and disorder when there is no organizational energetic force maintaining them in existence. Quite simply, without consciousness and a divine spark in the universe to create order and organization through divine will, all material would immediately revert to chaos, disorder, and disorganization. Without our divine light providing the blueprints for matter to follow, our souls and our bodies would not exist.

Based on the two profound truths above and based on the fact that we simultaneously exist as both aspects at all times, then it must be true that, as stated prior, we are simultaneously both our bodies and not our bodies.

We are *episomatic*. And we are profound and powerful beyond all imagination.

This is one of the greatest secrets kept in the Mystery schools across time and the biggest realization modern medicine fights tirelessly to prevent you from having.

EPISOMATIC NATURE IN ACTION

Our bodies serve as the interface for our physical and mental experiences. Because of this, and because of our inherent and innate ability to alter and create our own realities through changing our perspective and using our own creative divine will, we can sometimes experience this ability in a negative way. This can happen because we are either unaware of our own ability or we haven't been able to truly believe and trust in our own power. There are many ways in which this lack of trust, understanding, or conviction can affect our mental and physical health in negative ways, but first, let's take a look at ways in which we may have experienced a time when we were less than fully present due to external circumstances, and may have experienced what it is like to not be *fully in our bodies*.

BRAIN FOG

I will assume that most people reading this book have had, or will have at some point in their lives, some form of injury or at least some experience wheretheir physical and conscious interpretation of the world was shifted, altered, or muddied for a short period of time. (Not in the way you would think of in drug-induced states; that is another topic that we will not be getting into here). For some, this may have come from a concussion or a head injury. Others may have experienced this reduced consciousness while experiencing a severe infection or fever. For others, it may have happened while coming out of surgery after being put under anesthesia. All of these are prime examples of how you can experience this conscious clouding, and as a result, obtain a hint of subjective experience, proving that we are not just our bodies — that we exist in a perceptual form *above* our bodies, as *episomatic* beings.

If you've ever had one of these conditions or one of a similar effect, then you may have experienced something most commonly known as brain fog. Brain fog is different for everyone but is generally experienced as a splitting of the physical and the mental in a subtle but noticeable way. It's the realization that although things don't *feel right* in your body, and the way that you're perceiving and interacting with the world is noticeably *not right*, you still have the ability to objectively be *knowing* and *experiencing* that your sensations are off. You effectively see, from a higher vantage point, that your current experience, as seen through the seat of the observer, is not the normal experience you have in that same seat. This simple realization should not be able to happen unless we exist as our bodies and above our bodies at the same time and can experience both vantage points.

If we were just our bodies without our inherent episomatic qualities, then when we experienced, say, a head injury that caused a shift and our experience of reality dropped below its optimal level of function, then we wouldn't actually be able to recognize that we are functioning at a lower level. We would not have the capabilities necessary to realize that we are not interacting with the world appropriately. If we were simply a computer-based system with neurons firing in response to stimuli (like neuroscience would like us to believe), we would not have the capability of *knowing* we are operating at a lower level if our system is disrupted. Rather, we would take in the experience as it is, without context or question of experiential quality.

To an outsider, our mental and physical performance may be noticeably diminished, but to ourselves, from within the seat of the observer, we should not be able to experience that sensation unless we were episomatic beings with an expanded awareness above and beyond our physical bodies and possess the ability to compare the current experience with past experience accurately.

If you have ever experienced one of these situations or any other situation that has resulted in brain fog, then think back to those times in your life, and you will realize that you experienced that situation as if you were separate from your body. Like you were looking into the moment and at your sensations almost as an outside entity, realizing the sensations you were experiencing didn't *feel* right compared to what you knew they *should* feel like. Your brain had a previous memory of how you typically feel when interacting with the world, and there was a distinct, perceivable difference between this baseline and how you were experiencing it at that moment. This vantage point of conscious memory and ability to compare and contrast is unique to higher-level beings and serves as a direct experience of our episomatic nature.

In these moments, we instinctively know how the world *should* look and feel if all things were clear and appropriately represented based on our previous experience. When there is a change to that perception, even a very subtle one, we know it right away. We shouldn't, but we do.

NEAR DEATH EXPERIENCES (NDE's)

A further demonstration of our *episomatic* nature comes from near-death experiences. In these instances, many individuals will report experiencing themselves floating above their bodies and watching the entire scene of what is going on during this temporary separation of soul and body. In many of these reports, when questioned, the individuals have often been able to recall specific details of conversations and events unfolding and taking place around them during this time of separation, such as the actions and conversations between doctors and nurses in the operating rooms. Despite not getting much media attention, reported NDE cases and these phenomena are very well documented.[6]

These are both examples of our episomatic natures and serve as evidence that we are expressions of divine energetic archetypes that inhabit our bodies with the right conditions that allow us to interact with the physical world as long as these conditions are maintained. When these conditions are no longer present and we detach from our bodies, we still exist with all our consciousness maintained in another form.

Between these two properties — our true, divine, archetypal light and energetic source; and our somatic, material, physical structure — we come together to form our true expression in this world as dualistic, *episomatic* beings.

---

[6] If you would like to read more about experiences like this from first-hand accounts, I would suggest two fabulous books titled "Dying to Wake Up" by Dr. Rajiv Parvi, and "Heaven Is Beautiful" by Peter Baldwin Panagore.

Just as Jesus Christ was divine and materially human at the same time, we, too, are divine and materially human.

We are divine light, and we are material bodies. This, I believe, was the true teaching of Jesus and the message he was trying to convey, and why his message was deemed so dangerous that he was put to death.

Once we truly realize this, we will no longer need priests, rabbis, and prescription pill pads as go-betweens. We will be free. Divine beings can no longer be controlled by fear of deterioration of our physical bodies because we know we are eternal, regardless of our bodies.

That is true empowerment.

EPISOMATIC IMPACT ON HEALTH

The understanding of the duality of our existence is important moving forward for health and medicine because we need to circle back to a place where our spiritual and divine beings are integrated into one universal understanding. Our spiritual health can no longer be considered separate from our material and physical health. It is the division of these two into distinct categories that has led to a supreme amount of suffering, ignorance, purposefully misleading agendas, and misinformed campaigns that have spanned hundreds of years and plagued so many generations.

Once we collectively decided that we should pursue health and medicine as strictly logical beings, through empirical means only, we attempted to view and understand our physical bodies without acknowledging or pursuing the understanding of the divine energy source that animates them. We ignored the very thing that creates life, so medicine became the study of disease instead of the study of life. It's like trying to understand a gas-powered engine without acknowledging the flame that creates combustion.

Instead of conceptualizing human health as it truly is, we have divided these ideas and placed the divine spark in a philosophically constrained religious idea. That aspect of ourselves has been secluded to a place of which we have no immediate access or understanding of. It's saved for religious doctrines and relegated to only be relevant inside our churches, synagogues, and temples, but never relevant or real inside of the temples of the Religion of Science, such as hospitals and doctors' offices. This castration has led to no true study of this intimately important part of our physical existence and a glaring lack of understanding of how it is intrinsically linked with our health.

This divide has resulted in a schism that, over time, has grown into a giant chasm between our understanding of our physical health and understanding of our spiritual health. To move forward in our healthcare practices, we need to draw a bridge between these two separate categories and realize that not only are they connected, but they are, and always have been, intertwined and enmeshed in every imaginable way. To move out of this time of medical ignorance, we need to look at the physical body as the other side of the same coin of our spiritual body. We also need to open our eyes to the obvious manipulation of both sides of the coin in our physical reality. Only once we begin to accept this truth will we be able to begin to build an adequate understanding of ourselves and our true nature in this physical world, as well as our true nature and purpose in the divine realms in which we concurrently exist.

We must work with both these realms to create lasting and genuine health and happiness for ourselves and all individuals on this planet as a whole. We must come together in consciousness, as well as action, to move ourselves out of the darkness and into the light.

Out of chaos and into order.

Out of disease and into health.

The conscious awakening that has been occurring over the last 100 years has increased in noticeable intensity recently. This global awakening has allowed the framework to be laid out so we can begin to understand our spiritual and divine selves more pragmatically and begin to use these understandings to rewrite our ideas of health and move into genuine alignment with the divine, as well as alignment with the laws of our material bodies.

During this time, discoveries and scientific advancements that we have undertaken as a species have provided us with more powerful tools to be able to measure and perceive our physical reality to the point that we have now progressed to a place where the discipline of physics at its highest levels, show no separation between the consciousness and the physical realm. Physics has demonstrated that the energy that pervades and fills every single space in this cosmic reality both affects and is affected by our consciousness. This intimate give-and-take relationship, which has now been demonstrated in the emerging field of epigenetics, has been shown to affect the mechanisms of regulating our genetic and cellular expressions on a second-by-second basis to most effectively allow us to interact and respond to the environments we are in, both internally and externally.

Between the two disciplines of quantum physics and epigenetics, we have been able to demonstrate and begin that daunting task of understanding a scientific framework that illuminates a link between the conscious realm and the material world in such an unquestionable way that we are led right back to the elephant in the room that has still yet to be addressed.

This elephant has been there all along, but we are now staring at it face to face, and it is becoming impossible to ignore. This elephant is the understanding that our physical, conscious, and divine selves are *all equally entangled aspects of our human existence* and the existence of the cosmos. Every single one of us is made up of the totality of the cosmos and is actively and unquestionably both experiencing and creating the universe in a delicate, intricate, and beautiful symphony of information, energetic, and physical exchange.

Now that we have begun to understand the impact of our conscious perception on our physical reality and how it can be altered in specific events or situations, I would like to bring some attention to the idea of reality itself and what it *really* is.

CHAPTER 9

THE HOLOGRAPHIC PROJECTION OF OURSELVES

If you haven't read the book "The Holographic Universe" by Michael Talbot or heard any other versions of the Holographic theory of reality, then I absolutely suggest that you explore this topic further if it interests you. I may even recommend you put this book down right now and buy Talbot's book because the information inside it had such a pivotal impact on my life that I couldn't imagine where I would be if I had never read it. That being said, if you still have this book in your hands, then I'm going to assume you aren't rushing to your car, so I will give a brief explanation of the premise here.

The Holographic theory states that, due to the irregularities and unexplainable aspects of our physical reality, the only way to reconcile these anomalies is to understand that we are actually living in and experiencing a holographic projection, not a physical reality as we perceive it.

A hologram is unique because every portion of it, when divided, contains the information of the whole. So, if you were to take a holographic image, cut it in half, and then shine a light through the one half of it again to animate it, even though it is only half of the original image, the whole image would appear. This pattern remains no matter how small you cut the pieces; the only difference is that the further you divide it, the less detailed the image becomes. You lose only the precision of the picture. This can be used to explain the fractal nature of our physical reality but also can support the idea that within us, we have atoms and molecules that carry the information of the entirety of the cosmos. So, we, just like a holographic image, contain all the information of the whole.

Meaning our DNA may contain the blueprint to all that has and ever will exist, buried deep inside every one of our cells.

Using this framework, the holographic theory states that we are in a holographic reality, and physical reality is not actually physical at all. Now, I can understand if you are new to this, it may sound a bit preposterous, but remember Newtonian physics demonstrates that we, and all other material things, are nothing more than trillions of atoms held together by electromagnetic force. But what does an atom consist of?

Well, much of an atom is actually empty space. In fact, it is said that if you took all of the actual dense physical mass of all of the atoms of the entire universe, they would condense down and fit into a sewing needle. This means that 99.9999999999… percent of all material in existence and all matter in the universe is empty space. So perhaps the idea that reality isn't all that physical after all may make a lot of sense.

But if material isn't quite physical, and we are just experiencing a holographic projection of reality, then are we just holographic projections ourselves? And what would that even mean?

Well, let's take a look.

ARE WE HOLOGRAMS?

Have you ever noticed how people can look different on different days? I'm not talking about wearing different outfits or trying something new with their hair — they *actually look* different on a core level in a subtle but noticeable way. I'm sure some days look in the mirror at a chunk of unruly hair, or at one of your eyes all puffy and think, "What's going on with thiiiiiis today?!"

I remember making jokes or comments a few times in my life after a day of not sleeping very well that I was so tired that even my hair was tired. Those were days when the normal flow, curl, and wave to my hair wasn't present, to the point where it seemed like the blueprint of my hair just wasn't right that day and seemed a bit distorted. Do you think that perhaps there could be a little bit of validity to this? I sure didn't — not until I read the holographic theory.

We are not static beings, but perhaps this idea goes further than the dynamic exchanges we discussed in previous chapters of balancing internal and external environments with pieces of matter that have existed elsewhere in the universe. Perhaps this is true on a more subtle and profound level, in that every single day, we have slight variations to our physical and conscious forms based on the quality and clarity of the holographic projection of us being received and presented in physical matter each day.

If we really are an energetic projection, then it is likely that depending on our conscious, energetic, and unique frequencies on a day-to-day basis, we can likely have disruptions, alterations, or changes to that projection — perhaps even on a second-by-second basis. It could also be likely then that certain things could increase the clarity and strength of this projection while other things may reduce it. Unobstructed vs. obstructed projections. This could be the true holographic reason why everything from thoughts, sleep, food, moods, and emotions can have an instantaneous and measurable effect on our physical bodies, the way in which we are currently experiencing reality, and why your spinal alignment and nervous system communication as the receiver of the holographic signal may be such an important factor to your overall health. This could also be why we show and present to others slightly differently on different days. And if we are tuned in with ourselves, we can even pick up on it.

I have two prime examples from when I was able to actively notice this in individuals routinely. One was an ex-girlfriend, and the other was a roommate. Depending on the day, I would notice that their eyes would look in slightly different directions from the center, while other days, they looked completely straight on. What if this was a distortion, a wrinkle in their energetic blueprint projected into their holograms, showing as a slight disruption of their bodies? For them, the major things that had an impact on bringing them back to the center were sleep, being adjusted, and not going out on a bender the night before. Perhaps we all have these disruptions and variations daily, and maybe someone close to us may know one or two that they have noticed in us before. Maybe we are all flashing in and out and changing at such a high rate of speed, in such a dynamic way, that we appear solid and consistent but may have innumerable variations that express themselves off and on in our projection that, if looked at long enough, may be able to be predicted and measured.

PLATO'S THEORY OF FORMS

Plato had a famous theory that I believe encompasses the principles of holographic theory and the possible idea of us being projected in a dynamic and changing way based on some perfect form of us existing somewhere else, i.e., the perfect blueprint for the holographic projection. This is called the Theory of Forms.

In this theory, Plato believed that there existed, in a different dimension of reality, some form of perfect existence in which all things that exist in our current imperfect world are preceded in this alternate dimension where they exist in a perfect state and are used as the blueprints for the imperfect representations that exist in our own dimension. An easy example to conceptualize this would be the idea of a perfect circle. In this perfect dimension of reality, there exists the true and real version of an absolute perfect circle. No flaws. No approximations. Perfect. Because this perfect circle exists in this dimension, the idea of it exists within our dimension of reality and our collective consciousness and can be projected here into the physical reality, but only as a close approximation and never the complete, true version.

Despite the idea of a perfect circle existing in our imperfect reality, it is, in fact, physically impossible to make a circle that is 100% perfect in our material world. Even in our digital world, if you zoom in far enough into an image, the perfect circle begins to pixelate into straight lines and edges. So, even though a truly perfect circle is an impossibility in this dimension, the perfect circle in the realm of *forms* does exist. Because it exists in this archetypal dimension, it can project the idea of that circle upon our reality where we can get ever-increasing approximations, but never a truly perfect and infinite circle. Regardless of the idea being projected as accurately as possible, there will always be some alteration to the code as the signal passes into our reality. The result is that the actual circle that is created is in lesser proximity to the original, perfect form. However, certain variables within our control may impact how much information is lost in that projection.

Combining the Theory of Forms and the Holographic Theory, we can entertain the possibility that the realm of perfect forms is actually the divine realm of God, in which we all exist as perfect divine entities, and the projection and approximation of our perfect divine selves is what is manifested in the physical world we are experiencing. So, despite our existence in an eternal, perfect state in one alternate level of reality, our physical selves are an imperfect approximation of our divine forms in this one.

Despite our trying, we can never reach perfection simply because the material world is, by definition, imperfect. Even with this apparent separation, this concept still begs the question: What can we do to increase the clarity, precision, and intensity of our projections to bring us to the closest approximation of our divine selves here on earth, even if we can never be fully and truly perfect in this material projection? And what is the mechanism through which we are projected here?

It is possible to think that from this divine realm, an energetic signal that is constant and pure, which represents us in our true, perfect totality, is somehow beamed down into our bodies, and in turn, our bodies have a receiving system that can integrate, interpret, and then project the information to create the image of us in our reality. When it enters this physical reality and is transmitted to our material bodies, some of the perfection and detail of this projection is lost through the nature of being translated to organic material. Though this may be an unavoidable fact, we may have some control over how much of that signal is lost and to what extent we can take steps to reduce it. If this is all true, or at least possible to be true, then every single day that we are alive, we are potentially a walking representation of our unique divine signal of perfection, and our actions, habits, injuries, and nutrition may just dictate how clear or distorted that signal currently is.

If we ponder the physics of signal transmission through any medium, we can conclude that, as the signal travels from the divine realm to the material realm, there are ethers and mediums through which this signal passes that are out of our control. The signal's ability to transmute through these areas, with or without blockages or disruptions, represents the purity of the signal we receive and the part of this process that is out of our control. Not only is this portion of the transmission out of our control, but it may also be truly unknowable as we do not know where the signal is being sent from in the first place and what mediums it has to pass through before we receive it. Nevertheless, when considering the purity of the signal, we know that up until the signal reaches our energetic bodies, we have little to no control over the amount of signal that is preserved and received. However, once the signal reaches our energetic and physical bodies, this represents the border in which we begin to have control over what quality of signal can be expressed through ourselves and where our personal responsibility is initiated.

This is where practices such as proper nutrition, sleep, exercise, and chiropractic can play an unbelievably important role in opening the energetic pathways for the signal to be received and perpetuated. Think back to the discussion of the kundalini energy through the spine and the roles of fats as insulators vs. highly efficient and conductive body compositions as means of effectively distributing the signal to the cells of the body.

Another effective treatment that works along different energetic pathways would be acupuncture, which is based on pulling energy through stagnant ley lines in the body to increase proper energetic flow and distribution. Despite working on different energetic pathways, both chiropractic and acupuncture share a similar basic purpose and philosophy: to remove physical, energetic, and chemical blockages that inhibit and alter the flow of energetic information, life force, and signal transmission within the body.

As demonstrated in the above chapter on the Kundalini, when we have a clear and undisrupted path of flow up and down the spinal cord out into organs and tissues, then we have a high-quality signal and clear antenna into which our divine signal can be first received, and then accurately distributed throughout our entire being. When we are in alignment, we are connected to the divine realm, and we can receive and project the clearest and most accurate signal of our divine expression of form into the physical world. By reducing interference, we allow for the highest quality of transmission and become the closest proximity to our divine selves that can physically be possible in the material world.

This is, and should be, the goal of all forms of medicine and all avenues of medical research if the human experience were properly understood. Unfortunately, it seems that this is an area of medical research that is under a supreme level of suppression and denial instead, being delegated to the dusty and forgotten corners of medical interests because no pharmaceutical drug in existence would increase your energetic clarity because all medication are forms of poisons that undoubtedly take away from it. Luckily, the chiropractic profession, along with other natural healing paradigms, has been able to maintain this wisdom and continue to work to honor the body's innate ability to heal and push back against the "outside-in" mentality of modern medicine.

As it turns out, there are even more subtle ways in which we have control over this holographic projection of ourselves outside of the ones detailed above. Sometimes, simply knowing how our body is designed to function replaces the inaccurate stories we have been told and can remove *conscious* blockages, resulting in a surprisingly clearer projection simply because it is no longer distorted by the *energy of fear* or the subconsciously programmed limiting beliefs.

Let's take a look at how we can stop our educated minds from interfering with our innate minds and how changing our programming and individual stories can potentially change our lives.

CHAPTER 10

EDUCATED VS INNATE BRAIN

The title of this chapter tips its hat to a famous quote attributed to a man named B.J. Palmer, the developer of chiropractic and the son of D.D. Palmer, the creator of chiropractic. BJ is the person responsible for bringing chiropractic into the world of scientific and objective study.

Nicknamed "The Developer" for his role in further developing the idea his father created, B.J. Palmer believed that our educated, rational thought and our bodies' innate intuition and abilities were sometimes at odds with each other. He famously told his students, "Your educated brain gets in the way of your innate brain."

When I was first presented with this piece of history in the early months of my graduate program, I initially found this phrase rather questionable and counterintuitive. After all, at that time, I was neck-deep in the process of developing my educated brain, so it almost felt undercutting and insulting. After years of ruminating on this idea and the experience gained by venturing out and starting my own practice right after graduation, I can say that this phrase has grown more and more relevant in my mind and experiences every single day — especially when we come to the astounding realization that our education may have been more of a purposeful indoctrination than genuine teaching of truths.

The process of education is really just the process of learning and integrating elaborate stories about certain topics into our belief systems. We are told stories that are said to be true by people who are supposed to know best, and we are taught to believe them and regurgitate them like it's our job, because it will be. We are tested and scored based on our ability to retell these stories as close to the original as possible. The higher your education, or longer you spend studying a topic, the more intricate those stories become and, often, the more certain you become of them and the more you consider yourself an unquestionable authority in that field. After all, that is part of the structure of the indoctrination program. This may be helpful to hold and maintain this place of authority in some ways, such as when we are in an objective position looking at the events or concerns of another person who is coming to us for our help and we are the ones acting as the experts in the form of a doctor, surgeon, lawyer, mechanic, insurance agent, etc., or any form of observer separated from the event; but can be hurtful in others. Like when you are the main character INSIDE the event, experiencing it. Your expertise, though still helpful when interpreting your own events, can also be harmful if left unchecked. As once said by Robin S. Sharma, "The mind is a wonderful servant, but a terrible master."

When you are the main character in the event, you become a subjective actor. When you are a subjective actor, your educated mind may interfere with your ability to see the information objectively and may even begin to interfere with the abilities of your innate brain and body. You may inadvertently use your education to override your innate function and send your body into a spiral of subjective information disguised as objective information, effectively hijacking your innate processes along the way. Nowadays, we have so much access to information that this phenomenon can occur for any individual, regardless of having formal education in the topic or not. I know a lot of people who are a heck of a lot more educated on a certain condition than their medical doctors because they are the ones diagnosed with it, so they have studied it relentlessly. Formal education or not, information can be helpful and empowering or dangerous, depending on how your subconscious brain uses it.

Take someone who has been trained to recognize the signs of a heart attack, such as a doctor or first aid responder, or someone who has had a loved one have a heart attack, for example. Their teacher will have drilled into them what signs and symptoms to watch out for and be forced to memorize the typical sequela, or progression of a heart attack, and what symptoms would be associated with it.

From an objective standpoint, this is very useful information and arguably, everyone should have some training in this topic, but what happens when this information is applied to the subjective experience of an individual? What if this person happens to be a very nervous person with a habit of worrying and overthinking? Or maybe they have a diagnosis of generalized anxiety disorder. Now, we are met with the phenomenon that science wishes it could bury and pretend never happens. The mental and emotional response of the person, coupled with the knowledge of what to expect from the event, creates an environment in which it becomes very easy to manifest the sequela of a heart attack in the individual's mind, *especially* if they have a thorough education on what they should expect to see.

This is a daily problem for thousands of people who have become extremely nervous about their health and extremely good at creating the signs and symptoms of emergency health scenarios by unintentionally hijacking their conscious minds and forcing them to override their innate minds. The worst part is, as previously mentioned, with the advent of the internet, you no longer need any formal education in any of these conditions; WebMD places all the anxiety-provoking information right at your fingertips. This ability to read information and instantly create a mirage version of it in our subjective reality results in the true and honest terror associated with the real condition as your body creates the sensation of the symptoms correlated to the condition. This has been exacerbated and purposely exploited for power and profit over the last four years and has now been cultivated into a tried-and-true psychological weapon.

The highest expression of this condition would be called *health anxiety* (formerly known as hypochondria); however, most people experience some level of this hijacking throughout their daily lives, which affects their decisions and actions throughout the day. Health anxiety has become the norm over the last four years, and the individuals who have been lucky enough not to suffer from this condition are now seen as the weird ones.

Let's look at an example of a respiratory illness in the family of the common cold. Now, imagine you were an individual who lived out of town on a farm with no access to the Internet, TV, or radio.

Over the last four years, if you began to experience the symptoms of a cold, you likely would have made some tea, maybe even a hot rum toddy, and rested for a few days as the symptoms passed. However, if you aren't lucky enough to live on a farm completely disconnected from the rest of the world, and over the last three years, if you began to experience symptoms of a common cold, your response to these symptoms was likely clouded by a sense of sheer and utter panic. This panic, along with the news telling horror stories about the progression of these symptoms falsely packaged to look like well-intentioned warnings, likely would have led you away from a hot rum toddy and warm bath and closer to dialing 911 and spending the night in a cold sweat as you awaited your impending doom.

As you frantically went to the local government website to study the list of common symptoms to watch out for, they likely began to appear in you, along with the ice in your veins of a person who truly thinks they are dying. Every single one of these new symptoms added to the panic you were experiencing. Panic mixed with propaganda and knowledge — what was sold as education on the condition — created one of the most stressful and illness-provoking environments in our recent history.

Dr. Bruce Lipton, the most prominent scientist and researcher responsible for bringing the field of epigenetics into the world, states, "You cannot be in fear and growth at the same time." This means that the more scared you are, the less efficient your immune system is, and the less efficient all systems in your body function. Reduced immune function means increased symptomatology and increased severity of whatever infection or virus you are fighting. But what if you knew nothing about the news and the panic around this cold? What if you just faced it like you have faced every other cold you have had in your entire life: with total ease and trust that your body knew what to do? Likely, you wouldn't have had nearly as intense symptoms. Even more likely that it would have passed much quicker than it did and would have never made it into your mental memory bank as anything more significant than the countless other colds you have had in your life.

Knowledge is power, but knowledge without wisdom and a properly controlled mind can also be more dangerous than beneficial. As hard as it was, we needed to be reminded of this truth.

Fear and growth are mutually exclusive. Fear shuts down the body's natural healing and growth mechanisms and places the body under chemical and emotional duress, which not only changes the function of our immune system but also changes the genetic blueprint currently being activated within our cells. Fear is helpful in short-term situations. However, prolonged experience of fear is one of the major contributors to disease and tissue distress in the body. Even short-term fear has been shown to have a massive effect on the immune system, causing immunosuppression almost instantaneously, but long-term sensations of fear are linked to detrimental and far-reaching health conditions like cancer, heart disease, and autoimmune disorders, to name a few. Fear itself is the absolute worst thing someone can allow themselves to experience if they want to maintain a highly functioning immune system and an accurately projected signal of themselves. Fear, when faced with a global pandemic, should be the absolute last thing a government that is really out to help you should be pushing. Unfortunately, it is instead the most commonly used tool to force support for political agendas because scared people are easier to manipulate and control.

Scared people buy products they are told will save them.

Scared people provide $1.7 trillion to a single company in just one year.

Scared people ignore all logic.

Scared people don't ask questions.

Fear, mixed with a rudimentary level of medical knowledge and a highly funded, immersive propaganda machine, creates a perfect breeding ground for hijacking our body's natural function by consciously overriding and interfering with a system that is thousands of years wiser than we are, and forcing it to follow our short-sighted instructions instead.

This practice has led to whole industries of chemical anti-inflammatories, decongestants, and fever-reducing medications — to name a few — along with an entire multi-billion-dollar industry of injecting diseases to prevent diseases. It has also created a society in which we have been programmed since the day we were born that if we begin to feel any symptom at all, we immediately need medicine to fix it.

We need a hero.

Symptoms are the enemy, and medicine is the hero.

This belief has set the stage for the incredible lie that we have all been fed — the lie that we are helpless babies who need potions, pills, needles, genetic modifications, and saviors in white coats to help us through any crisis of health because our bodies are wholly unable to adapt and heal without them. You can't get to heaven without a priest, and you can't survive this life without the constant intervention of a doctor and his prescription pad.

These ideas and the whole paradigm they feed are based on and sustained by one thing: education through stories of all the reasons we are weak, delicate, deficient, and desperately in need of saviors because our bodies are *not enough*.

But what if all this information, all this education, and all these stories are based on lies?

Or at least a large part of them?

What if all this indoctrination has just forced us to constantly interfere with our body's innate function and constantly forced us to override our innate mind by forcing our bodies to follow our educated brain's advice instead of its own God-given wisdom?

How many times have our educated brains been wrong? I mean, all the data collected over the last three years has demonstrated probably one of the greatest medical and political blunders in the history of the world. Is that enough for us to learn from? Aren't we getting tired of being told that our bodies don't have the ability to do something without help and then finding out that the help has created more problems than they were claiming to solve and that someone else, somewhere in the world was able to do that very thing without the help prescribed? Aren't we tired of the most basic and natural things about being human beings turned into processes that are now medicalized and mechanistic interventions?

From birth to death, we have been convinced that we aren't good enough to handle these natural tasks on our own.

After all, shouldn't something like delivering a baby be the most natural thing in the world? Literally every human that has ever existed has come that way.

Every.

Single.

One.

So why has it become such a scary, intense, and mechanized experience with bright lights, epidurals, cold steel, planned C-sections, ample amounts of drugs, and forced inductions? It seems our educated brains have turned the most beautiful miracle of life into one of the most stressful and cold experiences possible, both for the parents and the beautiful baby.

A cold steel table, latex gloves, and a slap to the back. What a great first experience of this world ... *not*.

So, what else have we allowed to be unnaturally altered because we have listened to our educated brains instead of trusting our innate bodies?

The problem with our education is that most education tends to belittle and disregard the wisdom of our ancestors and self-evident truths that have been passed on since the dawn of human beings. The reason for this is the medical system and the academic system were purchased by private interests a long time ago, and genuine innovation is looked down upon in favor of strong and intelligent ways to perpetuate the interests of the groups in power. Along with private interests, by the design of the programs, education includes the training of ego, and current formal education has made it its mission to basically rewrite wisdom by destroying and disregarding the old and forcing adherence to the new. Nothing is held sacred unless it can make money for a long, long time — not the wisdom of ancient cultures or the wisdom of our modern grandparents alike. Any process, from birth to death, that isn't generating capital gains, needs to be.

This ego-cation does more than just that. It also has done its absolute best to eliminate and disregard the wisdom present *within* every single one of our bodies — the wisdom that has created *all of life* and maintained each of us in existence since the day we were born and since the dawn of time. The single force that maintains all existence and provides a blueprint for all living things to develop and heal without help or intervention has been disregarded by modern medical education as some antiquated and disproven *myth*. The original and perfect projection of life that we all receive and animates the entire world has been forgotten.

We have gone so far as to recently alter the genetic code of humans in an attempt to play God, and unabashedly stand superior saying, "We no longer need the intelligence of the innate, and we are now more all-knowing than our Creator."

Surprisingly, instead of this belief appalling the average human, there seems to be an abundance of people who are more willing to place their short-term and long-term health in the hands of billion-dollar companies who have proven time and again to not be trustworthy of such a high order, and that don't have the slightest idea as to the long-term effects of what they are selling, than place their trust in the power that made the body, to heal the body.

As a society, we are seeing a pandemic of our educated brains interfering with our innate minds at a higher level than ever before, and we seem to be losing access to the knowledge that *we even have innate brains.*

Despite the huge leaps we have made as a society in technology, we *must* be able to admit where we are still woefully lacking. And when we have any doubt, side on the decision to allow our bodies to do what they have done for thousands of years; whether that's burning off pathogens through a fever or naturally bringing life into this world. Our educated minds are only useful when they are *smart enough to know when they are not useful.* Our bodies are strong, our bodies are capable, and our bodies know what to do. We need to step out of the way and let them do what they know how to do best.

CHAPTER 11

ORDER OUT OF CHAOS

Plenty of varying topics are openly understood to have a connection with our health. As mentioned so far, nutrition and exercise are the most obvious and widely accepted; but there are also more controversial things we should consider.

I haven't always been an individual who believed that lunar cycles, or anything else in relation to astronomy, could have a significant effect on our physical bodies. However, on multiple occasions in my clinical practice, it has been demonstrated to me, despite my consistent refusal.

I first noticed the astronomical impact of lunar cycles on our bodies when I worked security at bars and strip clubs during my undergraduate degree. It didn't take long to notice the trend that working a full moon was going to lead to an eventful night. If you ask anyone who works at a hospital or as a first responder, they will undoubtedly tell you the same thing. Despite knowing this intuitively, as most of us do, I still actively refused to really consider any further implications of the planets' energies in our solar system having any direct effect on us, mentally or physically.

With multiple years of clinical experience now under my belt and having experienced some major astrological events since 2018, it is now, much to my unease, almost impossible for me to think that these events, along with the accompanying positions of the cosmic bodies and lunar cycles do not have a direct effect on us energetically, mentally, and physically.

THE CATALYST

It occurred to me while I was at work in my chiropractic clinic, on a day before a particularly powerful full moon, that as everyone entered my office with their own subjective "crazy" thing that happened that day, that some pattern was emerging. Along with these odd events, I objectively noticed their bodies were showing irregularities from their normal patterns — something about the day was throwing everyone off, and I could see it in their bodies as much as they could feel it. It seemed that, even though all these individuals were, for the most part, oblivious to this peak of energetic information their bodies were currently in the process of downloading and responding to, their bodies were very aware and responding through the manifestation of symptoms and tissue quality changes. Admittedly, this was the first time I ever considered celestial bodies to be relevant to evaluating my patients' bodies, but the pattern was so strong and consistent throughout the day that it became hard to ignore. I realized then that it was my duty in those moments — and every day before and since — to help their bodies integrate and adapt to whatever powerful energetic influx they were subjected to and assist their bodies in creating order out of chaos.

Inner Alchemy.

It was at that moment I clearly understood for the first time that my sole job was to become an *energetic catalyst* for my patients. Through my physical adjustments, the energetic interaction between my hands and their body, and our energetic biofields — which begin to interact at a distance of about 10 feet from each other (The Infinite Mind- The Science of Human Vibrations of Consciousness- Valerie Hunt)— it is my job to provide an appropriate, positive, energetic stimulus that their body can use to facilitate integration, and reorganization of their physical, chemical, energetic, emotional, and spiritual selves with the new information and experiences their body has received. It is my job to create an environment in which their bodies can integrate the discordant and disturbed signals they were experiencing as symptomatic ailments and allow their bodies to turn this heightened and displaced energy into positive signals in harmony within their bodies.

Chaos into order.

Dis-ease into ease.

Inner Alchemy.

Although this revelation happened on a day of very powerful and obvious energetic transfer, it made me realize that this is true every single day, regardless of the moon cycle, solar flares, or time of year. Furthermore, not only is it true in my profession, but it's true for every individual across all human experiences when interacting with another individual. Some may have a more obvious and direct influence on it for other people, but regardless of your awareness of it or the amount of people you interact with in a day, it is universally true for all of us.

We are all janitors of this world — every single one of us — and we all share that responsibility, like it or not.

This may not sound like a very glorifying job, but it is the most important responsibility we can ever be given. Not only are we the custodians of this planet and this reality, individually and collectively, but through our custodial duties, we are the collective creators of it as well. Being an active agent and creating order out of chaos, you become a conscious creator of both your reality and that of the collective. You also have more impact on it than you can probably imagine. You can change someone's day in an instant, and you may be changing the world as you go. "You never know how far reaching something you think, say, or do today could affect the lives of millions tomorrow" – D.D. Palmer.

Despite the magnitude of this power, to take this information and use it purposefully, instead of only focusing on how we can change the world, we must first look within and work at changing ourselves. How do we create our own *Inner Alchemy*?

SIMPLE, BUT PROFOUND

Have you ever tried to study, read, or create anything in a room that was cluttered, disorganized, or dirty? (Basically, my entire youth and teenage years.) A messy, disorganized, cluttered environment is very anxiety- and stress-provoking and a hard one to create in. The mess is a physical expression of the discoordination of energy in our lives strewn about incoherently.

Our external environments impact our internal environments and vice versa. Research shows that younger individuals with messy rooms may have a higher intelligence because it demonstrates a personality of thinking outside of linear terms, so though this may have a purpose in our youth and development, it is not a sign of intelligence or having your shit together as an adult. Conversely, it is often the case that adults often find themselves cleaning their space when they should be doing the work or project that has a fast-approaching deadline. This cleaning, while it may seem like procrastination, is an innate response to attempt to organize our external environments to help organize our internal minds, and often results in more streamlined productivity when the attention is finally placed on the bigger task. We may consider it procrastination, but it is our innate wisdom helping us organize our energy so we can more easily focus on completing the task.

Another example is cooking. It's enjoyable to cook in a well-organized, clean kitchen, but it can be an absolute nightmare cooking in one that hasn't been cleaned or organized in weeks. The feelings of ick we get in these messy spaces are a perfect example of how our internalized messiness can be projected onto others around us, and, despite our best intentions, our actions or words may be perceived as erratic and incoherent and may make them feel the same ick. On top of how others perceive us, if our internal energy is extremely disorganized, then our actual physical representation will also be disorganized.

Think about the previous chapter.

If we have a disorganized mental and energetic antenna, then the divine holographic signal will be expressed as disorganized.

This can sometimes still work for people like artists since part of the allure of their brilliance is the unhinged and unpredictable nature of their personalities, which then translates into the same in their art, but unless your disorganization leads to insane levels of brilliance and artistic creation, your unhinged personality traits are not helping you with your outward presentation, nor are they helping your performance, and internal feelings of ease and productivity.

YOU ARE NOT AN ISLAND

The reason I bring this up is that energy and frequencies, in all aspects of nature, are designed to harmonize and entrain with frequencies around them.

If you place 100 metronomes on a table, and start them all at different times, you will see that they will sync up with each other 100 percent of the time in a spontaneous process called *entrainment*. All frequencies in the physical and energetic worlds interact, and all frequencies affect each other. The frequency you are walking around with, whether that is calm, collected, passionate, hating, loving, organized, or frantic, will have an instantaneous effect on every other person around you, usually before you or they even say a word.

Your internal mind and energy will inevitably affect those around you and how others see you and feel in your presence, even if you think they are exclusive to you. It is an undeniable and unchangeable fact.

So, when people say, "If you want to change the world, start with the person in the mirror," they couldn't be more right. The person you are and the interactions you have are a result of the work you do to cultivate your energy into a magnet, hyper-attractor of the same energy you are giving off, whether you do it knowingly or not. By accepting and harnessing this power, you can clean up your own internal kitchen, which will effectively help to clean up the kitchen of every person you interact with daily. You again become a custodian and a creator. The mundane becomes profound, and suddenly, your work becomes very, very important.

As we walk through this world, every interaction we have and every single thing we do gives us the opportunity to either introduce a positive, harmonious energy of love, compassion, organization, forgiveness, and light into that situation or we can inject negative, dark, disorganized, disruptive, and dirty energy. The choice will result in the expression of either emotions of love, joy, gratitude, and harmony or emotions like hate, anger, blame, frustration, guilt, and sadness.

You can either give someone a Mr. Clean magic eraser, or you can empty your garbage can all over their counter.

Choose wisely because emotions are contagious, and if you ruin one person's day, they will likely ruin someone else's. You create a wave with every interaction you have that ripples far further than you could know. This is why it is said that no one remembers what you say to them; they remember how you make them feel.

If you make someone smile, they will spread that joy to others as well. You can create a smile train. We are all catalysts and have a bigger ripple effect than we can imagine.

So what's it going to be? Do you want to help someone clean or dump your garbage on their floor?

It may seem like I'm missing a third option here: leaving the place exactly as it was before you got there. However, this is a *fictitious* option and not one that is provided to us in any real-life situation. No matter what, even if it's a tiny granola bar wrapper or a small spot on the floor, our presence will leave some imprint in some way.

If we are involved in any situation — and because we are not inert beings — then by definition, our being there and our involvement, presence, energy, actions, and words will have an impact on the situation and everyone involved in some way or another. This is simply the laws of physics and human interaction. It is impossible for us to be a completely neutral factor in any situation in which we are involved or present, no matter how benign or seemingly unimportant that situation is or how small our involvement in it is. Even if we stood completely still and silent in the corner during an event, the act of standing silent would be judged and reflected upon by everyone else involved.

The beautiful meaning of this is *your presence means you matter.*

Your presence makes you an active creator, and your actions, inactions, words, or silence are a choice and will have an effect somehow or another. You being present or absent, and what you do in either of those scenarios will change the ripples that leave it.

This undeniable and unavoidable truth means that *we have an undeniable and unavoidable responsibility* at all times in every situation to try to provide an energy or stimulus that helps bring that situation and everyone involved in it closer to order and further from chaos — closer to love, and further from hate, hurt, and fear.

Grace over guilt.

Forgiveness over spite.

Ease over stress.

Order over chaos.

Inner Alchemy.

YOUR MISSION, AND YOU HAVE TO ACCEPT IT

I understand that for some individuals, this may sound like a lot of unwanted responsibility, but just like we have the responsibility to eventually get a job, pay taxes, and take care of the children we have, we cannot run from this responsibility either.

Even the attempt of inaction is an action. Face it: everything you think, feel, say, and do impacts every person around you.

We can no longer afford to be selfish.

It's time to take responsibility and consciously perform our duties of creating order out of chaos. I hope that the information ahead will help in this endeavor because even though the human body and the mystery of human health may seem at times to be an inconceivably confusing and complicated pursuit, there is an extreme amount of elegance and order in how we function. We just have to learn to recognize the patterns and cycles our physical, mental, and energetic bodies respond to and provide them with the tools to do so in the most natural and unimpeded way.

The more we learn, the easier it is to recognize and actively accomplish our work of Inner Alchemy.

CHAPTER 12

OUT OF OUR HEADS AND INTO THE MOMENT

We have all heard the very sage advice to get out of our heads and live for the moment at one time or another. However, whenever we attempt to integrate the task of living in the moment versus endlessly sifting through the current of thoughts and never-ending events passing through our minds each day, it comes down to simply choosing one of two options: allow them to flow freely past us or to fixate on them- because let's face it, there is no way to make them magically go away.

Despite our best intentions and all the yoga classes and meditation courses we can attend, it's likely that if you are anything like me, you still have a hell of a time not fixating on them. In fact, trying *not* to fixate on them makes you fixate on them even more.

But what effect does this decision really have on us? Is it just a nuisance to get stuck in the thought-wheel, or does it scientifically affect us, and on what level? Well, it turns out that the answer is explained quite well in quantum physics and prompted one of the first experiments that proved our reality is much stranger than we have been led to believe.

Fixate or flow is the equivalent of the difference we encounter in quantum physics between observing and not observing a particle. When a particle is observed in laboratories, it collapses from a waveform of possibility into a finite, measurable particle. The simple act of observing the wave causes it to condense into a particle every single time, but when it is not being observed, it returns to a waveform.

Similarly, when we observe or fixate on a situation, whether that be an event in the past, a thought, or a symptom we are experiencing, we collapse it from the wave of possibility into a finite thing. It is the figurative opening of the box of Schrodinger's cat: We create an outcome. We create a physical conclusion or a finite idea about a thing that existed prior as the possibility of many things.

Let me explain.

In quantum physics, as mentioned above, it has been demonstrated that the simple act of observation crystallizes and materializes a waveform into a particle as soon as it is observed. This is, not surprisingly, called the *Observer Effect*.

These groundbreaking experiments have shown that particles *always* exist as a wave when they are not being observed, but as soon as the conscious observer enters the picture, they condense down into a particle — almost like a subatomic game of hide-and-seek.

This is important because this experiment was first conducted on particles of light (photons); however, the same effect has since been repeated and demonstrated with *whole atoms*.

Humans and all other solid objects appear to the naked eye as a solid unit. Despite this appearance, we are made up of hundreds of trillions of these entities (atoms) interacting and being held together in a cluster through electromagnetic forces. We are a cluster of atoms held together by electromagnetic energy.

So is everything else.

Despite being a cluster of countless trillions of these atoms, it still must remain true that the properties that exist in one atom must exist in all atoms. Therefore, those properties must exist throughout and within the whole. This is important when it comes to understanding where we put our attention and how real we may be in a physical existence.

It also, as you will see, matters where we place our attention and thoughts daily and what effect that may have. After all, we just showed how observing an atom collapses it into a particle and creates an outcome — and we have also discussed how thoughts and emotions can affect us physically and create positive or negative health related outcomes. We are now beginning to dive into *how* that happens on an atomic and subatomic level — where the weird gets weirder.

On any given day, we are presented with a substantial amount of internal and external stimuli. All events that take place, either in our environments or our minds, cause reactions in the form of the conscious production and experience of thoughts and emotional states responding to each one of these stimuli. Every time this happens, and every second we spend ruminating over the event that just played out, it is a second in which we are *observing* the situation — collapsing the waveform into a particle. That particle is an event we then replay in our heads — sometimes spending hours or even days thinking of ways in which we would or should have done something differently. We spend this energy on maintaining the outcome in a particle and finite state.

This can also present in someone's life as a fear of having a disease, ending in that person constantly fixating on a symptom they keep experiencing and, over time, collapsing the wave of possibility and creating the outcome of the disease. Through the power of your conscious attention, you are enhancing the experience and confirming the presence of the symptom or disease. Your fixation prevents the symptom from reducing back into a wave and potentially disappearing instead of maintaining the outcome of the symptom in its physical form. Through subjective experience, you are constantly collapsing the waveform into a particle — the particle being a symptom — and, eventually, your symptom(s) into a measurable illness or disease.

These are just two examples of how we are constantly living in a state of collapsed waveforms. We have taken from the infinite realm of possibilities and created a repeating observation of a single possibility. This is the power of fixation, especially when driven by the compounding power of fear.

Alternatively, when we are truly living presently and are dedicated to being in the moment, we are consciously choosing to be living as a waveform. We experience the ebb and flow of life as a waveform. This means that we flow with ease; that when emotions and events happen, we acknowledge them, let them go, and move past them. With each event, for a short time, we condense into a particle for that moment to acknowledge the event, as we should, but the key is that then, when we let it go, we open back up and default back into a waveform.

Waveform consciousness represents a state of ease. The continuous compression and expansion allow us to interact on a neutral plane with all these experiences with acceptance and ease, all while maintaining a neutral and open consciousness.

This is the ideal state: The trained and earned level of neutrality and bliss that is spoken about as the famous state of *nirvana* and the goal of all Buddhist teachings. This is the place we all wish to be. The bad news is that it is very, very difficult to achieve full-time. The good news is that even if it can only be achieved for a few moments a day at first, those are moments of true bliss and possibility. Once you achieve this state, it becomes easier to revisit it. It is a learned state and a skill that can be practiced. Regardless of how difficult this may be at first, the pursuit of this state is very important for our overall health and happiness. This is the state of ease, and with ease comes health.

So, when an event, worry, fear, or memory reaches our conscious level, we can view it as a wave of energetic information and acknowledge it but make a conscious effort to allow it to pass through us without taking hold, or we can let it grab us and sink its teeth in until we obsess over it long enough that we create a self-fulfilling prophecy. I'm sure you have noticed, as I have for myself, that when you continue to fixate on something and hold it in your mind and focus on it, that thing tends to grow in your mind and become your experience. This is the basis of the book *The Secret*. We attract the energies we put out, and we create what we place our focus on.

So, be conscious and careful about what you focus on.

Say you wake up with a tickle in your throat, and you cough a few times to clear it. If you spend the rest of the morning focused on that cough or focused on the fear of getting sick that has locked into your consciousness, you will find that the urge to cough and the sensation will continue to magnify over and over. You will keep clearing your throat and making yourself cough because of that mental fixation. Your throat will become raw and sore because of the forced coughing. Eventually, if you can't let this go, your throat will be sore, and you will continue coughing. You have created the outcome present in your mind and therefore, it is now present in reality.

Alternatively, if you find a way to distract yourself with something totally different, perhaps with a book just like this one, and you don't attach an emotion to the sensation of the tickle, you may find that half an hour later, you haven't coughed a single time, and your throat feels normal. This is possible because you have allowed your body to stop focusing on the sensation and thus allowed the particle of possibility to shift back into a wave and open to a different outcome.

Our conscious awareness of events, and emotions responding to those events form the conscious observation in which we condense all forms of possibility down into the particle, material form. We create the outcome in the reality of the world that we fear or focus on, or we open it back up to the realm of infinite possibility and commit to the flow. This is the power of Nirvana.

INNER ALCHEMY

all forms of possibility down into the particle, material form. We create the outcome in the reality of the world that we fear or focus on, or we open it back up to the realm of infinite possibility and commit to the flow. This is the power of Nirvana.

CHAPTER 13

SUBTLE SIGNALS ON THE BODY

UCLA biophysicist Beverly Rubik published a study in 2002 titled *The Biofield Hypothesis: Its Biophysical Basis and Role in Medicine*[7] that demonstrates how the human body responds to minute electrochemical and electromagnetic signaling in ways not yet well understood in current scientific literature.

Rubik suggests that the human body subtly but measurably uses the various electromagnetic signals in its environment to help regulate its internal environment and physiological processes. These signals can be strong or weak, according to our understanding of electromagnetic field generation, and likely encompass varieties of signals and wavelengths that we have yet to discover or understand. Essentially, all electromagnetic signals within our external environment provide information that our internal environment and

---

[7] This information can be found on page 66 and 67 of *Electric Body Electric Health: Using the Electromagnetism Within (and Around) You to Rewire, Recharge, and Raise Your Voltage* by Eileen Day McKusick.

cellular processes are designed to respond to, whether we know it or not. (It will be important to remember this study when we get to Part II of this book.)

Putting this in context of everything we have discussed so far and the appropriate ebb and flow cycles of our body based on signals around us that are as subtle as changes in temperature, sunlight, and the electromagnetic charge from the sun (to state a few of the ones we know of), we can begin to see a dire problem when man-made signals that are of much higher electromagnetic intensity are being placed in our environments without us knowing it, and at ever-increasing numbers.

In 2020, Elon Musk sent more satellites into the atmosphere than the collective total of satellites ever sent to space before. Everything is electric, and everything related to sending and receiving satellite and cellular signals of any kind must be, by definition, pumping out a huge amount of information in the form of electromagnetic signals, as well as signals containing the information that is being sent and transferred, directly to the environment around it, and therefore directly to us.

Whether the signals we are responding to are overt and obvious signals, such as the presence of light, which prevents the natural production of melatonin in our body, or more subtle signals, like the information coded in every text message that moves through our bodies en route to its intended target, it is clear that current science cannot even begin to fully grasp the possible impact these various subtle but powerful signals have on the human body. Despite not having any mainstream coverage on this topic or even any genuine consideration of it, it is highly probable that the effects of the signals we are bombarded with daily in our energetic environment may be as obvious and measurable as the natural environmental signals that trigger seasonal changes inside of us (more on this in Part II). It may be probable that these new synthetic energetic signals are interfering with our innate responses to natural environmental signals, creating disharmony between us and our external environments.

Think about this for a second. If every single text message, phone call, or television signal carries with it the information coded to present its intended message onto a screen or out of a speaker, what if that coded information, to some small degree, is being read and interpreted by the body on an energetic level? It is clear that our bodies are negatively responding to high levels of electromagnetic frequencies, as demonstrated by the work done in virology labs, in which scientists have been able to *actually create viral particles* from living human tissue when they expose it to high levels of EMF radiation; but what if the information carried within that EMF radiation was also having an impact on the cellular expression of the body from a more subtle level? This is the level of thinking and consideration that we should be using to investigate these topics if we want to truly improve human health and reduce human disease processes in the future.

How do these frequencies affect us? How does the specific information inside these signals affect us? Do they only affect us on a cellular level, or can they alter our emotions, too? Can they alter and impact our perception of the world?

In a study performed by the Heart Math Institute in California, individuals were placed inside a room that conducted a coherent electromagnetic frequency calibrated to be similar to that of the earth's natural electromagnetic frequency. When test subjects were placed inside the room, they were asked control questions about how they felt emotionally and physically while sitting in the room when the coherent frequency was still active (they did not know of the frequency, nor did they know the intentions of the experiment). During this time, the subjects reported feeling normal and calm, claiming no ill effects or discomfort whatsoever. That was until the electromagnetic field was suddenly turned off — without the test subjects knowing.

Once the experimenters turned the coherent electromagnetic field off, effectively dropping the internal electromagnetic field of the room to a very low state — much lower than the base frequency of the earth — the subjects began to feel uneasy and anxious within minutes. This continued to progress rapidly, and some even felt ill and nauseated.

The sudden change in their emotional and physical states led the subjects to unravel mentally. Subjects began crying and became angry, frustrated, and unstable. Some even started to have full-out spontaneous nervous breakdowns. The change in the electromagnetic field they were subjected to triggered an internal response resulting in the sensation of incoherence and an experience of genuine panic and anxiety. The electromagnetic energy in their immediate environment instantaneously altered their emotions, physical sensations, and mental states.

* * *

The study above demonstrates that when our environmental electromagnetic frequency is altered, it alters our internal emotional and physical experience. One could also assume that sometimes, when we have these experienced states of reduced coherence in our bodies and minds, it could be due to our internal triggers, like memories or emotions, instead of external triggers — I am sure often happens completely unrelated to external factors; but what if the electrical signal in the external environment we are in becomes altered or the sudden change actually does have a lot more to do with our emotional experience than we think?

It's possible that unbeknownst to us, the electrical charge around us changes, or a piece of energetic signal data passes through us with negative-coded information, resulting in a disruption to the flow of information from our brain to our body and a bombardment of new subtle information is passed through us. Perhaps this shift in stimuli and communication of new information and energy effectively alters our internal communication and creates a feeling of unease or incoherence that we perceive as an emotion or a negative thought. Or what if they are both effectively the same process, but one is from an external source, and the other is from an internal source? Either way, we have all experienced the sensation of moving from coherence to incoherence, and we all know how quickly that shift can happen with seemingly no real reason. I have had many instances where I was feeling incredibly good and grateful, and just at that moment, out of nowhere, a negative, stress-inducing thought came into my mind and changed my internal experience on a dime. The importance of this is understood when we refer to the information in the previous chapter. How we feel and our emotional state can have a direct impact on how we perceive the environment. So, whether the negative stimuli come from an obscure energetic event or a real-life one, the change to our internal dialogue and experience creates a change to our outer world experience instantaneously. An example of this happened while I was writing this segment of the book.

Before I began writing, about 20 minutes earlier, I was sitting in my vehicle reading another book (I often get flashes of inspiration to write while reading from other authors). At that time, my internal subjective experience of the moment and my environment was great. It was fantastic, actually.

I was parked in the parking lot of my childhood elementary school in an area that was familiar to me from years of living within a few blocks from this spot. I was filled with positive memories I had from years of attending this school and playing with my friends in that exact spot. All these stimuli were working their magic on my emotions and tickling my nostalgia. This precise place in the world brings me a lot of joy and positive emotions because it activates happy memories for me, and it is a place I often visit for that exact reason. It was a beautiful sunny day, and I felt blessed and grateful.

Then I received a text message.

The text was from a long-time patient of mine who was reacting very strangely to a treatment given to her by a massage therapist a few days prior. The patient sent me pictures of a rash that had spread all over her face and body, causing welts and swelling in her lymph nodes that started hours after the massage and had progressed rapidly. Despite this not happening directly to me or to anyone in my immediate family or close friend group, the moment this information came into my energy field and conscious awareness, I felt an immediate drop in my own energy and an evaporation of my sensation of happiness. Immediately, I began to feel somewhat distressed and uneasy. It was like all the energy of the sun and the environment around me was just taken away. Like someone flipped the switch from coherent to incoherent energy.

Now, this may seem normal and unremarkable at first, but what really stood out about this experience when looking at it retroactively is that not only did I *feel* internally distressed, triggered by my empathetic response to my patient, but I actually *began to feel distressed about my environment* as well.

The shift in internal energy resulted in me beginning to have incoherent and unhappy thoughts about my environment — the physical spot that I was in that I, just minutes earlier, was expressing so much joy and appreciation for. I was now noticing the parking lot was busier than I wanted, and the kids playing in the park were being too loud, and the sun was covered over by a cloud. Just minutes prior, I was in total calm, peace, and enjoyment, but following the message, I became restless in that exact same environment, having a completely different experience. I began to mentally notice all the reasons it was a bad spot to read and debate whether I should drive to another location instead.

I began to feel anxious about being there. The sun was literally now completely covered by clouds. I began to think about other places I could go to park that would *feel* better. I began internally and externally analyzing everything in a negative light and even turned on my vehicle to drive away… Until I realized what had just happened.

I experienced what I was planning on writing about in real time.

So, I stopped and looked at it from a new perspective, the one you see on these pages. My internal electromagnetic frequency shifted due to information that entered my conscious and energetic field. Because of that shift in electromagnetic frequency, my experience of the world instantaneously changed.

I changed my world and the very place I was in *because my electromagnetic field shifted*. This time, it was because of a change in the electrical environment due to real-world information, but how often does this happen to us because of a change in an electrical field around us without us even knowing the reason? Could the information that was coded into that text message have traveled through my body and interacted with my subtle, energetic, and cellular bodies as it made its way to my phone? Was this a dual interaction?

I believe this experience confirms Rubik's research discussed above in a more subtle way, showing that both our internal *and* external energy fields must remain high and within an appropriate range to maintain coherent, happy, and healthy emotional states. I believe our energy fields are susceptible to change based on electromagnetic signals that pass into our energetic and conscious fields, just as they are to electromagnetic fields that exist in our external environments. Both have a direct and immediate effect on our thoughts, emotions, and cellular tissues. When our internal or external electromagnetic fields shift, it results in incoherence in the communication of our bodily systems and affects every aspect of our physical and subjective experiences, all the way from our emotional experience of the world down to the intrinsic and subtle cellular processes that happen second by second to keep our body functioning and healthy. Altered levels of electromagnetic fields result in altered experiences of the world around us and, more importantly, altered emotional and conscious states, which results in altered mental and physical health.

Our experience of the world consists of our response to internal and external environmental signals. Coherence in conscious life is the action of our minds and energetic bodies constantly interpreting and communicating with the stimuli we receive to create an appropriate relationship with the environment around us and an appropriate function of the tissues in our bodies. This constant communication between our body and the queues it receives from the external environment, as well as the information and cues it is constantly receiving from our internal conscious and subconscious environments, dictate our level of experience of the world we are in and calibrate the precise way in which we respond to it.

Second by second, every single day.

We are barely starting to understand this relationship in nature and within the human body itself. Even though the study of this relationship is an ongoing process with huge amounts of data and insights coming forth yearly, it is still quite elusive to mainstream consideration. Much information has been censored and buried about this topic to protect the interests of many agencies, such as the mountain of data demonstrating the irrefutable dangers of the 5G grid on human health. This data is suppressed because the purpose of the grid, in the eyes of the stakeholders who have paid for it to be forced onto the streets of every country in the world, far surpasses any concern about the health implications.[8]

If we as a species have only recently begun to understand there is a positive charge from a flower and a negative charge from a bee that works in a symbiotic electromagnetic relationship to attract the bee to the flower and that this pattern of subtle attractive forces has been coded into all parts of nature since the beginning of time, then how can we be so egotistical to think we could be anywhere close to understanding the true extent of the subtle relationships that exist between all the vast, and countless organisms in nature, including ourselves.

All organisms transmit and respond to electromagnetism from every part of nature, every second of every day. Even bacteria are driven by electromagnetic detection and attraction. Electromagnetic signals are the basis of organic life,

Solid objects appear to be solid because of the magnitude of the electromagnetic field pushing against our solid bodies when we pick them up or run into them. All things are just energy, and all forms of energy are, at their core, just information. Our subjective reality, and the reality of all living species, is a dance of subtle pushing and pulling forces between each organism while interpreting and integrating the bundles of information they carry with them.

---

[8] If this is a topic you are interested in researching deeper, then you can find an extremely through and eye-opening analysis of the effects of the various man-made electromagnetic fields on human health over the last century in the mammoth of a book called "The Invisible Rainbow: A History of Electricity and Life" by Arthur Firstenberg.

If there are subtle energies that can be emitted from blades of grass, trees, or flowers strong enough for our bodies to recognize and respond to them in ways that can have instantaneous positive or negative effects on our physiology, then imagine what effects the significantly stronger electromagnetic signals that are being sent out from our electrical devices, may be having on our bodies on a second by second basis. Doesn't it seem like a good idea to figure this out before we add to the electromagnetic soup we are already bathing in?

The relationship between human health and electromagnetic fields, both internal and external, is yet another huge blind spot in mainstream medical science. We must open to this reality and begin to advocate for the necessity of understanding this relationship properly in future scientific pursuits. If we don't, we are running the risk of vastly harming our health and ignoring the high likelihood of measurable and predictable negative health outcomes due to our natural responses to unnatural amounts of energetic and informational stimuli.

CHAPTER 14

THE POWER OF WORDS & SYMBOLS

We may, at first, consider words to be just inert, unimportant tools used to communicate a thought; however, the true power and purpose of words is a highly esoteric and profoundly important topic.

Though for some, this information may seem too grandiose to consider for others reading, it may already be common knowledge. I presume that if you are reading this type of material, you must fall at least somewhere in the middle. As with many topics in this book, my goal is to bring the esoteric and hidden to the eyes of those who are on the path of seeing but haven't quite found all the answers yet. The power of words, at their true core, serves as a basis for all the ideas written about in this book. It represents how things we use and interact with every day can play a more significant role in creating our experienced reality than we once were told.

The words that you use, whether in the form of thoughts to yourself (internal affirmations, running daily internal dialogue, or recurring emotion/thought patterns) or the words you use externally

169

when interacting with the rest of the world via all forms of communication, including verbal and written, have a dramatic and direct impact on the manifestation of the world around you. In fact, the words you use in all these different channels collectively join with your conscious perception of their definitions and your emotional experience of them to become the forces that create your reality and, thus, form your experience of the world. Words are creative forces, and every single word is like a small magic spell being cast out to the universe. This can be summed up in the term, and arguably most famous *real* spell, "Abracadabra." The term *abracadabra,* which dates to the second century, loosely translates to "I create what I speak." Despite this term being one not often used in our current society outside of parody, it encompasses an idea that remains wholly accurate in all forms of communication, whether we know it or not. —Even the word *spelling* comes from the origin of using words to create a spell.

Through spelling, you are piecing together a spell, and just like Abracadabra states, whether we are aware of it or not, we create what we speak.

The power and effect of words are overlooked more than any other facet of the human experience that we have direct conscious control over. As individuals and as a society, as stated in the previous chapter, we must begin to explore these realms of science that are pushed to the periphery by the mainstream because these tend to be the areas that carry the most reality-altering truths.

The power to use words to create and manipulate reality has been known by the select elites and mystery schools for thousands of years. If we want any chance of understanding our place in reality and taking back control of our own lives, we must begin to first understand and then reclaim the power that words have over us. Once we do this, we can begin to unlock the secret power within them and purposefully begin to harness it for ourselves.

By understanding the true potential of the magic that exists within spelling and the energetic influence carried and transferred in each word, every single one of us can consciously, strategically, and purposefully have a better ability to create the world around us by consciously selecting the words we use in communicating with ourselves and others— and what we allow into our minds in the form of music and media. This means being aware of the phrases we utter, even when they may just be colloquial sayings you think may not mean anything. Or worse, when we make joking statements that, if looked at through this lens, could be detrimental spells unknowingly cast.

* * *

On any given day, we make multiple statements in which we identify ourselves with certain qualities or certain things by using words to relate our state to a particular event or feeling. For example, when someone comes into my office and says, "I'm broken," or "I'm falling apart," or "I have pain here," it's a declarative statement that's affirming and identifying for them using these magic words, which little by little convinces reality to begin adhering to the words they speak. Recently, I was walking through the mall when I heard a teenage girl say, "Fuck my life; I will literally die if we do that." Yikes.

There's a vast difference between the examples above and when someone comes into my office and says, "I'm experiencing pain here" or "There's a few things that haven't worked themselves out yet, but I'm feeling better every single day." And in the case of the dramatic teenager, she could say, "Fuck off, I do not want to do that," and land the same effect without the negative energetic implications. You can still be cool. Just be smart with your words. Be cool *and* smart.

Re-framing the way we speak reframes what we experience. We rewrite the spells that are winding together to create our lives. We grab hold of what we can actively control and become the pilots. But what about words spoken by others towards you? Can those also have an impact on creating your reality?

Absolutely.

If you let them.

"I AM WHATEVER YOU SAY I AM"
-Slim Shady

Think for a second about when someone receives a medical diagnosis. Often, a diagnosis has an instantaneous effect on how a person feels physically, mentally, and emotionally, but it can also seemingly instantaneously change how they feel about themselves *conceptually*. The diagnosis becomes an instantaneous edit to their life story that shapes everything not yet written and colors everything in the past and present with a new light. Healthy to sick, strong to weak.

Instantaneously.

The typical progression of subjective experience in the time immediately following the diagnosis for that person, depending on the severity of the diagnosis, usually transitions through a phase of despair, during which that individual quickly begins to identify with the diagnosis, both consciously and subconsciously, visualizing the worst-case scenarios in their mind. It becomes part of their story, *and often, it is the story that maintains the diagnosis in their lives, even years after many of the symptoms have been resolved.* These individuals now live with a consistent record playing on a loop in their subconscious mind telling them that at every given moment throughout their day — even when they are feeling happy and distracted — there is always a threat they should remember. Never let your guard down, and never be truly happy because a scary disease is hiding just around the corner, and today could be your last.

This loop plays in the background of their mind like a faint record on repeat playing out of the vacant spare bedroom of a house, and even when they try to tune it out, it is always there to constantly remind them of their condition and that at any moment, things could get worse.

When they are happy, the loop plays.

When they are sad, the loop plays.

When they are feeling pain, *the loop plays.*

These words and this diagnosis become a self-fulfilling prophecy because they constantly reidentify with them. Through the conscious and the subconscious minds, the energetic patterns inside of that individual eventually start to *become the diagnosis.* The spell that was cast becomes fulfilled. Interestingly, this can happen regardless of whether the diagnosis is accurate or not.

Let me repeat that: *You can create the condition even if the condition isn't present—the* magic of words.

An interesting example of this happened recently in my clinic. I had a young female patient who was recently informed by her doctor that she was experiencing a miscarriage despite her not even knowing she was pregnant. The doctor said her hormones were all over the place because she was undergoing the process of spontaneously losing the baby. Following the appointment, she became emotionally distressed. She stated that she "felt the loss of life" from within her and started experiencing all the symptoms of a miscarriage, including stomach pain, spotting/bleeding, sadness, and rollercoaster hormone levels. This triggered a deep depression and a very unpleasant physical state for the patient in the weeks following the news.

Just over two weeks later, she went back for her follow-up visit, but this time, she saw a different doctor as her regular doctor was on holiday. The patient told the Doctor she was struggling mentally and physically as a result of the miscarriage, but the doctor looked confused. The new doctor asked her why she thought she was having a miscarriage, to which the patient recalled what her regular doctor told her on her last visit, and she had been spotting since. The interim doctor checked her medical file and declared that she was not suffering from a miscarriage, nor was there anything in her file or bloodwork to suggest a pregnancy whatsoever. There was no record of the incident or the conversation between the patient and the original doctor to suggest a miscarriage.

It turns out that her previous doctor read her the wrong chart two weeks prior, and all the symptoms, all the varying physical and emotional changes, including the spotting that this girl had experienced for two weeks, *were self-created by her subconscious* based on her expectations of the diagnosis given to her. The word *miscarriage* created a spell that resulted in all the associated symptoms showing themselves, even though there was no medical reason for them.

Events like this happen much more often than you would think. The *placebo effect* (a positive feeling or phenomenon of spontaneously healing based on the belief that a treatment or procedure will heal you), and the *nocebo effect* (a negative feeling or phenomenon of spontaneously becoming ill or experiencing disease symptoms because of a belief that a procedure, substance, event, or treatment will hurt you) are the two most scientifically and medically consistent outcomes that have been documented in all medical research. Unfortunately, because the only explanation can be that the mind has the power to heal without drugs or interventions, and the mind can hurt in the same way, this information is disregarded as "junk data" and ignored in scientific literature. Instead, media outlets use this insider information to drive fear and sickness while simultaneously denying our healing properties so they can instead feed you a stack of pills that barely work better than a placebo and pretend it's a cure. They piggyback on the healing properties of the placebo and place them into pills and potions, and the public is none-the-wiser.

But I digress.

THE PARADOX OF DIAGNOSIS

The placebo effect is a very well-known but incredibly ignored fact in the medical world. It accounts for roughly *30% of all improvements in clinical trials globally*. Yes, you read that right — roughly 30% of patients in any given clinical trial are *expected* to improve simply because they *believe* they are taking a drug or undergoing a treatment that is helping. All clinical trials must account for this percentage. When the trial is over, statistical tricks are used like sorcery to try and prove that a drug is better than the placebo, in which case it would allow it to be called a success and be marketed to the public.

Instead of studying how 30% of subjects in all clinical trials are expected to get better simply because they believe they are getting an effective treatment, the medical science world treats this as the fat needing to be skimmed off to access useful data.

Why?

Well because you can't patent and sell the placebo, so they aren't in the business of glorifying it. They are in the business of making money, and they do this by proving that their drug or treatment, regardless of the laundry list of side effects, can be even a few percent more effective than the placebo alone, so they can package it and sell it for a massive profit, all while denying that the ability to get better by conscious action alone exists. Fun fact: this same level of ego and ignorance resulted in geneticists calling 90% of our DNA "junk DNA" because they do not yet understand its function, and it couldn't be used in the CRISPR (Clustered Regularly Interspaced Short

Palindromic Repeats) research that they were doing with the Human Genome Project.

Imagine that. Imagine the most complex and efficient informational storage technology we have ever encountered, being deemed 90% useless information.

Make that make sense.

To add insult to injury, the beloved Human Genome Project, which I repeat, considers 90% of our DNA as junk *because they don't understand what it does*, is the program responsible for inventing genetic manipulations that could be administered through a needle to alter our DNA permanently. Convenient right?

Just saying.

SPELL CASTING IN EVERYDAY LIFE

Outside of the hugely overlooked negative impact of medical procedures and medical diagnoses on people (death by medical error is the third leading cause of death in the United States, titled "Iatrogenic Death"), our everyday words also have a largely overlooked effect on the energy we are casting out to the world, and the energy we are feeling within. This ties back to the topic we discussed in the previous chapter about changes in electromagnetic information coming into our subconscious fields and its effect on our emotional, physical, and energetic experiences — except what if simple words had the ability to also alter our energetic states when we read, heard, or spoke them?

To demonstrate this, I want to do an exercise.

Now, you may want to just read past this without participating, but I implore you to try something right now while you're reading this book that will allow you to experience what I am trying to explain in a very real and visceral way. Don't worry, it's for science.

I would like you to say these words out loud: *Hate. Fuck. Shit. Bitch.* Say those words and see the resonance that you feel in your body when you do.

Now, take a second to cleanse your energetic palate, and say the words: *Amazing. Beautiful. Grateful. Thank you,* and *You're welcome.*

Did you *feel* the difference?

Try it again if you have to.

I will almost guarantee that you felt two distinctly different effects inside your body. I also expect that outside of just the energetic sensation, you likely had two totally different conscious experiences with those sets of words as well.

When you spoke each set, you likely had a visual flash of either memory or situation in which those words would be relevant and related. The memory will be one that was coded with the information stored in the *emotion* of those words. Likely with the first set of words, you had a flash of a memory or situation that pissed you off, and you still haven't fully let go of it. Maybe even the face of someone specific to go with it. However, it's likely that with the second set of words, those negative emotions vanished and were replaced with a positive memory or picture in your mind, like a family member's smiling face, the perfume of your sweetheart, or a flower in a field.

Words instantaneously send a vibration through us and out into the world, which we pass on to others who hear those words, read them, or are part of that interaction. At the same time, we have an internal scene created that our mind and body use to complete the context of the event that we then respond to. Even if just for a split second, we create an all-encompassing event filled with emotion and imagery, which we use to identify and experience words by layering some form of personal context onto them. This is how we learn and distinguish sensations of emotions — by attaching them to events that define the experience of that emotion or word.

We learn through association.

By doing this, we can create an event of an experience instantaneously based on every single word that we say, think, read, or hear.

This has been one of the most profound realizations I have ever had, and it seems to be very clear evidence that we *actually can* create what we say.

Abracadabra.

But this pattern extends much further than just the words that we choose to think and speak. It reaches things we identify with as well as the image that we create of ourselves that we project to the outside world.

Every word, idea, or thing that we gravitate to and integrate into our overall appearance and physical representation impacts the collective bundle of information we convey to others — and that we become ourselves. For example, if you're wearing a shirt that has a negative phrase on it, like *sin, reject,* or *destruction, dead inside,* or any other word or phrase that comes with a negative energetic association, then you will, both publicly and internally, knowingly or not, identify with those terms physically and energetically. They will imprint on you in some way or another.

Your body is an energetic inkwell, and the terms you wear and identify with, imprinted onto you energetically, interact with you and your holographic projection. This may seem a bit hokey or too woo-woo for you, but like it or not, it's true. And if you have made it this far in the book, then it's likely you are a bit woo-woo, too.

I once had a Nirvana shirt that was one of my favorite casual shirts to wear. Nirvana is my favorite band, so of course, when I saw it, I bought it and wore it without question. It was a black, long-fitting T-shirt that said Nirvana in big, bold white letters and had a whole bunch of small writing wrapped in a spiral design in the background that I never took the time to read. I just liked how it looked, so I bought and wore it. One day, when I was taking it out of the dryer, I took the time to read the small print that was written inside the spiral pattern in the background of the shirt. To my surprise, *on that shirt was written every single one of the seven deadly sins.* This had literally nothing to do with anything Nirvana ever wrote or stood for and was definitely not something I wanted to have *imprinting onto me.*

I had been wearing a shirt for months that had the physical energies of all seven deadly sins imprinting onto me without me even knowing it! Yikes!

Needless to say, despite how rad looking the shirt was, I never wore it again. Regardless of how cool something is, I am not willing to identify with it or be in any way attached to it at this point in my life unless it is providing me with positive energy and raising my vibration. I have misidentified with enough shit over my life and done enough shit over my life that robbed me of vitalism that I am no longer willing to do anything that doesn't bring me happiness and positive vibes. Period.

Good vibes only. Legit.

If you are reading this and it still sounds silly or extreme, then I implore you to try and fully commit to just one month of actively choosing positive words and energetic associations at all times in the words you say, clothes you wear, shows you watch, and music you listen to. You will be surprised by the power of this change and the shifts in your life when you start to take conscious ownership of these decisions. When you start to actively look at the clothes you're wearing and the words that surround you, whether they're on pictures or posters in your house, on clothing, your favorite lyrics, or the stories coming out of the mouths of the people you surround yourself with, you will begin to realize just how much control we have over creating our environment and customizing our reality — and how much control we have actively given away by not paying attention until now.

Once you start sifting through the energetic spells you surround yourself with and the subliminal energies imprinting on you from those spells, you begin to consciously dis-identify with them and systematically begin the process of removing the crap in your life that you may have never realized was weighing you down. Then, instead of the negative identifications, you will consciously start identifying with positive words and positive frequencies. You will begin to strategically place them around you like positive, energetic satellites, and you will notice a very tangible shift in the energy you both give out to others and feel inside. You will change your energetic environment, which will change your energetic expression and, along with it, your energetic effect on others.

In case you still need more proof, some studies demonstrate the power of energy held in the written word. In these studies, water from a sample container was put into multiple individual containers, which were split into two groups. The containers for Group 1 had the word *love* written on them. The containers for Group 2 said *hate*. Researchers then used an eye dropper to place droplets of water onto pieces of glass from each container, and they froze them. To their astonishment, they found that the frozen droplets of water obtained from the *hate* containers froze in very chaotic and unorganized patterns. Whereas the droplets from the *love* containers froze into beautiful, crystalline, organized patterns, much like the snowflakes that we're so used to seeing in movies that fall from the heavens. Each snowflake was unique, but the ones that were imprinted with a negative energy froze erratic and disorganized, while the ones imprinted with a positive energy froze in beautiful, organized, and symmetrical patterns.

This study shows that the vibration and energetic information carried by a simple written word on the outside of a container has a profound and completely penetrating effect on the water inside that container. Now, given that we are essentially giant bodies of water, it is obvious that this pattern would also influence us, that the written words we attach to our bodies or allow within our environment must affect our own energetic and physical structures. So, choose what spells you allow to be cast on you from the words you associate with. No fashion can be worth that price.

WORDS AND MANIFESTATION

Let's dive a little deeper into this. Restated a simpler way: All words carry energy.

They carry frequency.

They carry power.

They carry the potential of the thing in which they represent and the context around that thing.

Each word has a unique frequency to it. It has a unique vibration that carries information into the world, much more encompassing than just the dictionary definition. It carries more than just what that word describes in each language in literal terms. It also carries with it the *essence* of the thing it relates to, which instantly colors the thing it is being used to describe.

A word like *power* carries with it the energetic signature and frequency that *gives* power, along with a myriad of examples of people and things we consider power*ful*. The same goes for words like *love* and *respect*, along with ones with more negative connotations like *delinquent* or *rebel*. Each one of these, along with every other word that exists in any language, are more than just letters placed together, but are packets of information that carry with them energetic currents of that which they are. Letters *spell*ed together create a *spell*.

Every single word in every language is a spell that creates a thing when spoken, read, written, heard, or thought. If I said *elephant*, it's likely that, upon reading the word, you thought of an elephant. That written word instantaneously created an elephant in your mental world that never would have been there at this moment had it not been spelled to you. Now, if I say two novel words together, such as a *fuzzy elephant* or *pink kangaroo*, it is likely that you have just created in the mental world the appearance of two distinctly new animals that have probably never existed in your mental reality before I spelled them into existence.

By combining four simple words that are part of your everyday vocabulary in two unique ways, I not only created new entities in your conscious minds but potentially created one or two unique entities that had never been there or been experienced by you before in any capacity. Simply by using words to project them, we cast a spell and create something completely new.

Abracadabra, once again.

Words not only have the power to create — they also have the power to invent new and novel things simply by applying themselves in a new order. And then they have the power to bring that thing into existence if the proper force and mental energy are applied to it. Every word is a spell, creating a thing in the mental realm. Just like the Divine realm discussed in the Theory of Forms projects an image of us into the material realm; the conscious realm also projects an image of every thought we have, and it is up to us to use that blueprint to create it here in the physical realm. Everything in the mental realm can become manifest in the physical realm. Therefore, every word, whether spoken, written, or thought, can create and manifest its essence in the physical realm.

The extent of this power and responsibility tends to become lost on most people. Even individuals who understand this concept, in theory, can sometimes have a very difficult time adhering to its practice in real life. However, if you can learn to have restraint and discipline, then you will begin to see that by using your words carefully, consciously, and pointedly, and by consciously selecting the words you use in all situations, you will begin to wield the power to literally write your own life. If you can think it, it can be real.

Once you learn to harness this power, you can take control of your life and your story. When you do this consistently, your life will become a choose-your-own-adventure novel in which you have full power over deciding what each situation in your life means to you. You may not be able to control *everything* — there are far too many variables in this world to have total and complete control over all things — but you become empowered by knowing you can take every event and situation that is thrown at you and write the story around it for yourself. Furthermore, using the power of word spells, you can have a huge impact on how these events play out and which ones are presented to you. You can use words as spells to start attracting the situations you desire and cut out the old energies and frequencies that are no longer serving you, and you can go even further by actively deciding what you want to bring into this world, spell it, then create it with active energy and effort.

If simple word choice can be this powerful, then what other forces are having an impact on us that we may not even realize? More importantly, what other forces and tools can we learn to use to further control our realities and take back our personal power?

SYMBOLS, IMAGES, AND LOGOS

The responsibility of creating our realities extends further than just the words we use and the power held within them to manifest—we also need to be aware of the symbols around us and the huge amount of energetic information embedded with them that is constantly bombarding our subconscious minds.

Symbols and logos, such as the symbol a business or group decides to adopt to represent their brand, or the symbols used by governments to represent things like "stop," pack huge amounts of information and energetic input. A symbol is a carefully crafted image that represents the fullness of a certain thing, packaging a larger message than a single word would allow. So, if words are spells, symbols are sigils. And if you aren't familiar with what a sigil is, you obviously haven't done enough witchcraft in your life. (I joke, but it is a form of magic that embeds the energy of an idea, person, or thing into a simple symbol and is then used as a stand-in for that collective thing.)

I am sure you have heard the phrase, "A picture is worth a thousand words," and you likely understand this concept on a basic level. But have you ever considered this concept to stand true when it comes to something so seemingly inert as logos and symbols? After all, it's just a *swish*, isn't it?

On any given day, we are bombarded with symbols — recycle symbols, brand logos, vehicle badges, stop signs, religious symbols, social media notification badges, and so on. When you take a minute to notice, symbols are everywhere around you at all times. Just take one minute right now to put your book down, look within your visual field, and count how many symbols or brand logos you can see. In a quick 30-second glance around my living room, I counted 19 just from my single-seated visual field. Unless you are reading this naked, it's likely that even just looking at the clothes you are wearing, you are presented with at least three to four. Surprising, isn't it?

Now, if a picture is worth a thousand words, then how much information do you think these symbols are conveying to your subconscious and energy field at every single moment? Well, a lot.

Like, *a lot, a lot*.

You may not consciously realize it, but they are there, and they are influencing you in ways you cannot understand. Many symbols seem fairly basic, even inert, at first glance. That may be because you aren't consciously aware of their associations and base archetypal structures. Taking a closer look, you will see that almost all brand and application symbols/logos are embedded with one or more *archetypal symbols*. Archetypal symbols are the base structures that carry truths and ideas about the foundation of reality itself. The earliest written language was used based on symbols, and this pattern followed into Egyptian hieroglyphs and formed an alphabet of base structures that have been maintained to represent certain ideas to this day, unchanged. For example, look at the famous Freemason symbol shown below:

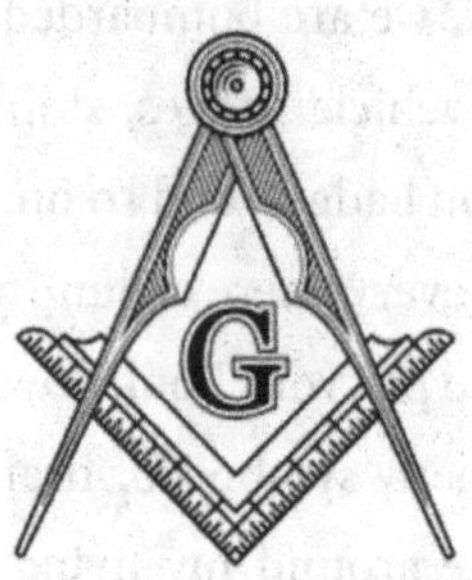

Outside of the immediate emotional reaction this symbol evokes in someone who is familiar with it, it also contains two main archetypal symbols: the upward-facing triangle and the downward-facing triangle. These base archetypes convey meaning in and of themselves much deeper than we know. In this case, one of the base meanings of these two archetypes combined is the hermetic principle "as above, so below." This symbol also carries the information of the divine trinity, duality, measured and right thinking (the 90-degree angle), and all of the esoteric teachings of freemasonry that are only available to the initiated. These principles are all packed inside this simple symbol.

On top of this huge amount of information being secretly conveyed, the masonic symbol itself, due to the power held within it and the reputation and history surrounding it, has itself become an archetypal symbol that other brands use to take advantage of its power to affect the subconscious minds of the public. Just look at the Apple App Store logo, for example.

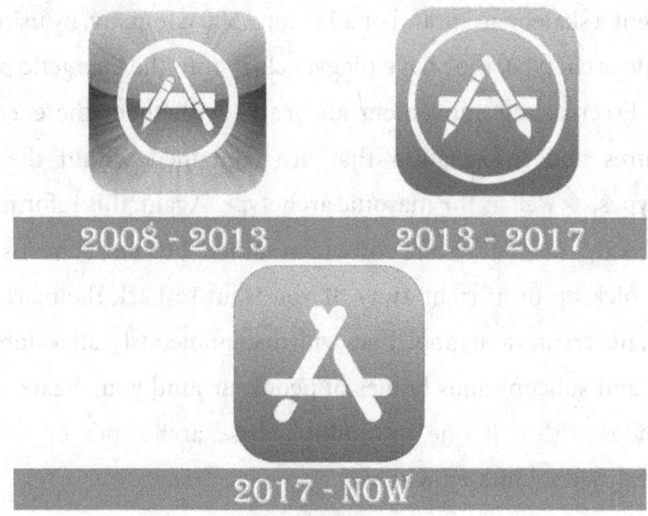

This is the layering of information that is contained within all symbols and the entire focus of the study of symbology, and a large portion of the study of esoteric and occult wisdom. Information is coded and placed in plain sight to affect the subconscious mind of the people who see it without them even knowing they are being influenced.

The same method is used when someone speaks in parables that are only intended to be understood by the ones with sufficient background knowledge on the topic to decipher them. This is why Jesus started his parables with the phrase, "For those that have ears to hear, hear that…" meaning that for most, this will be misunderstood, but for the wise that know, they will grasp the entirety of the meaning.

My task for you is, over the next day, to take notice of how many logos and symbols for seemingly unrelated things use a variation of the masonic symbol archetype. Even if those logos are supposed to represent a skateboard brand or a Fortune 500 company, by using the masonic archetype, they have piggybacked onto the energetic power of the Freemasonic movement and carry with them the energetic signatures and information that are contained within the base archetypes, as well as the masonic archetype. Again, this information isn't readily noticed by our conscious minds, but our subconscious minds pick up on it right away. If you want to hack the marketing game and create a symbol that will instantaneously stick into the minds and subconscious bodies of people around you, create a logo that hides within it one or multiple base archetypes or another powerful symbol hidden within it.

Once you understand symbols and their power, you will never look at them with such indifference again. On the other side of this, once you learn to see and interpret symbols, you will be able to see just how much they are used to manipulate and control our minds without most of us even knowing it. More importantly, you will be able to break the spell they have over you.

If you can be an active agent in deciding what symbols and words surround you and how you use symbols and words in your own life, you will hold in your hands an amount of power over yourself and your world you may never have known to be possible. This is some of the most sacred wisdom that thousands have worked tirelessly to hide from you; but today, it's yours.

CHAPTER 15

BIOTENSEGRITY

In the early part of the 19th century, an important organ was discovered, but despite becoming recognized as an increasingly important network of tissue connecting all systems of the body and having an ever-growing array of functions, that organ is barely mentioned with more than a fleeting acknowledgment in current medical textbooks. In 2017, that mystery structure was officially acknowledged as the largest continuous organ in the body.

That organ is called the *fascia*.

Through the ages, when anatomists and scientists studied the body, it was often done in cadaver form through human and animal dissections. When performing dissections, it was common practice to remove the skin in the areas where you were working to better visualize the underlying muscles, bones, arteries, and nerves. When removing the skin, the anatomist would also remove the thick saran wrap-like connective tissue holding the skin to the muscle and disregard it, as it was very fibrous and difficult to see through. It wasn't until recently that individuals began to *actually look* at that connecting tissue as possibly being worthy of study. Lo and behold, it was. Does this remind you of the junk DNA we talked about earlier at all? The part disregarded as useless miraculously turns out to be incredibly important. Who woulda thought?

When scientists finally turned their attention to the material they previously thought of as garbage, it was discovered that under our skin is a thick, strong tissue that acts as a single, unbroken unit and wraps around the entire external surface of our body and also goes inside our abdominal cavity and surrounds all our organs. One continuous tissue that connects every organ in the body with our overall structure.

One unbroken system that covers and connects the entire surface of our body with the entire surface of all our internal organs and can be affected by our overall structure.

This tissue is called fascia. And it's *kind of a big deal.*

Despite being able to perceptually divide it up into different *fascial lines*, as thoroughly discussed and demonstrated in the groundbreaking book *Anatomy Trains,* it is a single unbroken tissue that plays a very important role in motion, sensory perception, proprioception, biomechanics, and pain. It's been estimated that up to 50% of our pain receptors are embedded in this tissue, which has huge implications for conditions like chronic pain syndrome, myofascial pain syndrome, and fibromyalgia, which we will return to in a minute.

The role fascia plays in biomechanics is best explained through the concept called *Biotensegrity*. According to Biotensegrity, everything in our body is held together by a series of balanced tissues under tension, and a change to the position, alignment, or biomechanics in one area of that system will affect all other areas of the system. Like a drawbridge held up by pullies and cables in every direction, perfectly balanced. If any one of those pullies becomes too taught or too slack, it can change the structural integrity of the bridge.

I explain it to my patients like this: Think of a military-style bed sheet tucked in tight at all corners. Now, if you take your hand and go to one corner and crinkle up some of the sheets into your hand, you will see that every other corner must untuck slightly to accommodate. This sheet is your fascia, and this is the effect of biotensegrity on the body. Every minor change to the integrity of the body's alignment or balance of structural symmetry causes changes to other areas of the structural symmetry. As the entire body is connected, it is simply impossible for a disruption of alignment or function in one area of our body to not affect all other areas of our body in some way.

As a young, budding chiropractor, the first office I opened was a room in a local gym. Beside me were multiple physiotherapists and practitioners of other modalities, but I was the only chiropractor and the only vitalistic practitioner. I got along with most of the other practitioners quite well. However, I still remember one heated discussion I had with a neighboring physiotherapist that I still, to this day, cannot wrap my head around. She argued that if she had injured her knee, as an example, the change to the biomechanics in her knee *wouldn't result in any other biomechanical changes elsewhere.* She stated there was no science to demonstrate her injured and altered knee function would have an impact on her hip function, for example, or foot, and definitely nothing above her waist. Excuse me, but ... what?!

I stated that, by definition, a change to the biomechanics of her knee would unquestionably result in changes in force distribution and biomechanics in her hips, feet, spine, and so forth. It would result in unquestionable changes to the way her whole system distributed force while walking or doing any other exercise that required knee function to be involved. This is a fundamental truth in not only biomechanics and biotensegrity, but also all forms of structural engineering. It blew my mind how this base level of structural understanding and interconnectedness of the biomechanics of the body could in any way be argued by a physical health professional, let alone someone who is supposed to be the *authority on biomechanics of motion*.

Unfortunately, this was not the last interaction I've had with trained professionals in the health, fitness, and medical industries who seem to have completely missed the boat in understanding the very systems that they are supposed to be the experts in.

WHAT ELSE DOES FASCIA DO?

Further implications of fascia extend far beyond just simple movement mechanics. In chiropractic, we have a check that we do in our routine evaluations of our patients to look for biomechanical distortions in the neck, or subluxations, that directly affect the biomechanics of the rest of the body, all the way down to the feet. This is shown by something called positive cervical syndrome. To perform the check, we have the patient lie down on the table. Then, when a patient is lying in a prone position (face down), we evaluate their leg length. From there, we have the patient turn their head in either direction. If turning their head in one or either direction causes one of their legs to become shorter, then we have a positive cervical syndrome.

What did we demonstrate? We demonstrated that if they have a structural alteration, misalignment, or subluxation in their necks (cervical spine) through the interconnected system of biotensegrity (the sum of the balance of all the muscles and ligaments, and fascia as the bedsheet), the altered structural integrity of the neck is resulting in compromised biomechanics and tension all the way down to the heel of the foot that became shorter. Put quite simply: when that person turns their head from side to side, their spine and hips shift, and change the force distribution and balance of their structure, resulting in a change to the length of their legs if there is a subluxation in the vertebra of the neck causing a fascial distortion in the body. So, if someone's neck can affect the biomechanics of their knee, then their knee can affect the biomechanics of their neck.

This might seem rather inconsequential, but think about it like a structural engineer would. Your hips are your tabletop, and your legs are the legs of the table. The spine sitting on the tabletop is a broomstick and sitting above that is your skull in the form of a bowling ball. When the table is level, the legs are the same length, and the muscles holding the broomstick and bowling ball up do minimal work. Now, imagine you are doing a deadlift. The level of that tabletop becomes extremely important now that you are loading it. If you are loading your spine but have that neck subluxation causing a cervical syndrome, then if on your third or fourth rep of deadlifts, you turn your head slightly to glance at your form in the mirror, instantly your leg lengths shift slightly, and your tabletop tilts. This has now created an environment that results in uneven stress on your sacrum, your SI joints, your lumbar spinal discs, and your knees, and leaves you open to an unexpected injury. Simply turning your head and tilting the platform may put you at risk of injury, even if absolutely everything about your form is perfect.

This is just one of the ways people are injured doing things the same way they always have and why they walk into my office scratching their heads, frustrated as hell, wondering why, at this particular time, doing this particular movement resulted in an injury.

Knowing this and understanding the implications of biotensegrity, it is important to remember to consider *the whole body* when evaluating any injury, subluxation, a cluster of symptoms, or alterations in biomechanics. If you go to a medical doctor, or even many chiropractors or physiotherapists, and you tell them you hurt your back and point to an SI joint or the lumbar spine, you will likely get a small assessment of that area, but that area only. If you are lucky and have someone who really is using their head, you *may* even get an X-ray. But do you want to guess what that X-ray will be? It will be a lumbar spine-specific X-ray that will basically be a snapshot of the spot you pointed to on your back. No pelvic X-ray to evaluate if the tabletop is level, and definitely no neck and middle back X-rays to evaluate if there are any misalignments and compensational changes to the spine to accommodate the aforementioned biomechanical changes such as cervical syndrome. Basically, you would get a picture of one side of the bed sheet being pulled up slightly, causing discomfort in that area, but the radiologist and doctor would see a picture of a bedsheet lying *relatively* flat and say, "Normal X-ray."— Meanwhile, the crinkled part on the other side of the bed is being missed.

Your treatment will be directed specifically to the place of pain, and they will likely completely miss the underlying problem and cause of that pain. Pain is sometimes a symptom of a problem in the spot where you are feeling that pain. It is also, more often, a problem somewhere else, resulting in *the sensation of pain where you are feeling it.* Treating only the place of pain while not looking at the structure as a whole is like looking through a microscope and trying to see from the small tissue sample what the entire elephant looks like. Trying to fix one area of discomfort without evaluating the entire biomechanical structure of your spine and pelvis is like trying to set the table in an earthquake. You can spend all day setting that tabletop, but if every single time you turn your head, the top becomes unlevel and the foundation shakes, those damn cups are going to keep hitting the floor, over and over again. —And you are going to keep wondering what the hell is going on.

So, if you go somewhere for help with a knee problem and they also evaluate your hips and your entire spine up to your neck, don't look at them like they are an idiot — you may have just found someone who actually knows what they are doing.

Stay with them because you struck gold.

DIFFUSE PAIN AND FIBROMYALGIA

With the results of recent discoveries showing large portions of pain receptors embedded in our fascia, we have to look at chronic pain conditions such as fibromyalgia, myofascial pain syndrome, and chronic diffuse pain syndrome a little differently. Fascia is a living, feeling tissue, and the biotensegrity system is based on the balanced tension of fascia. If there is too much tension in one area of the body, or the body as a whole due to too many crinkles in the bedsheets, then it is likely this tissue will become inflamed and stressed due to chronic traction or stretching stress. If the tissue is under chronic increased tension, it will result in chronic inflammation. If this tissue has pain receptors within it, then it is logical to expect that those pain receptors would be sensitive to the sensation of stretching and inflammation and, in turn, register it as pain. It is also logical to think that this chronic stretching force and inflammation would result in chronic diffuse pain over many areas of the body and a heightened pain response when touched if the tension on the fascial tissue remains high for an extended period. This global increased tension and stretch stress would lead to global fascial inflammation and increased pain and sensitivity across the entire body. In other words, fibromyalgia—which translates directly to pain in fibrous tissue and muscle, and Chronic Diffuse Pain Syndrome— which translates to "you have pain all over your body, and we have no idea why, so we are naming it so it sounds like disease, and we can wash our hands of trying to find a cause." Loosely.

When evaluating chronic pain patients in my clinic, I have often discovered that their cervical (neck) X-rays show either a moderate to severe straightening of their normal curve or often a total reversal of that curve.

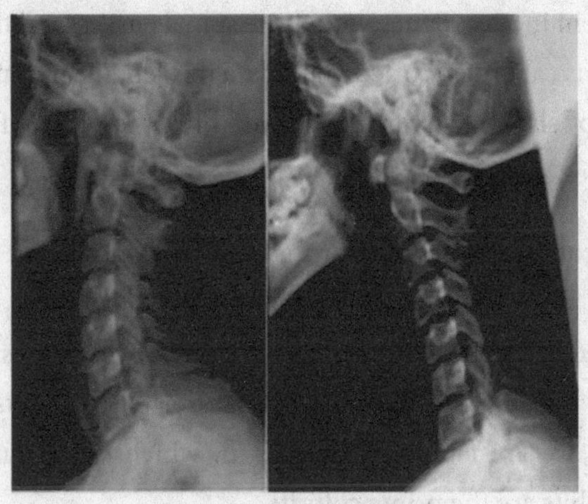

"Normal" Neck Curve (left) and Reversal

This is significant because as the neck begins to straighten, it puts tensile stress or *stretching stress* on all the nerves that leave the spine… which *is all of your nerves.*

When the cervical curve reverses, it increases that stretch on the spinal cord and nerves significantly. Just like muscle and fascial tissue in the body, nerves are a set length, and that length is based on that individual's size once they reach skeletal maturity. Your nerves, as they branch off from the spinal cord and leave the protection of the bony vertebrae around them, are anchored to the hole in which they exit called the foramina by connective tissue. The nerves are given a specific level of slack and held secure by tissue between the foramina and the nerve, keeping them within a normal limit of movement. Think of the nerve like a finger going through a finger trap — pull it in either direction, and the finger trap sinches up and stops it. When an individual reaches skeletal maturity, they typically still have normal spinal curves, so their spinal cord reaches a certain length at development in accordance with those spinal curves, and the slack on the nerves is calibrated to accommodate this length, and maintaining this level of slack is integral to maintaining the proper function of those nerves.

Any part of your spine can change shape and flatten out, which can cause this tensile stress, but it is most common and most exaggerated in the cervical spine, as shown above. Causes of this are most often injury-based, such as whiplash-related incidents; however, nowadays, we are facing more cases in which cell phone use and lifestyle habits are the prime culprits.

When the neck begins to straighten, it pulls on the nerves and stretches them since they are secured in place while exiting the foramina. If stretched enough, then the heightened stress on the nerve can change the firing capabilities of each nerve and lead to not only pain, but decreased overall function of those nerves and decreased function and health in the organs they are feeding. Remember that the nerves are electric. Stress on a tissue causes a change in the electric charge or signature of that tissue. Change to the electric signature of a nerve or the tissue directly surrounding it results in an alteration of that nerve's ability to transmit electricity, as well as the speed of electric transmission, aka a change to the function of your nervous system and its ability to respond to information. However minuscule these changes may be, their effects can add up to an overall global reduced function of the system.

Reduced function leads to dysfunction.

Dysfunction leads to dis-ease.

Dis-ease leads to *disease*.

Studies on the global effects of an altered cervical curve on overall bodily health and function, as well as its possible connection to fibromyalgia specifically, are starting to be conducted; however, the importance of spinal alignment and spinal health continues to be a blind spot in modern medicine, despite the obvious physiological implications. For that reason, just like an increasing number of aspects regarding your health, it is up to us to educate ourselves and pay attention to it.

Find yourself a practitioner who has the skill set to understand and evaluate your system *as a whole unit* first, taking into account your structural alterations and tensile changes *before* you turn yourself into a science experiment and begin taking the gamete of loosely prescribed medications in an attempt to chemically alter the effects of a physical problem.

CHIROPRACTIC SCIENCE TO THE RESCUE

The information on fascia and nerve tension causing diffuse health problems is new but groundbreaking. It adds an extremely important layer to chiropractic science and will play a significant role in allowing individuals to understand how their bodies function, why they hurt, and what to do about it. However, I would like to take a moment to turn our attention to the most fundamental science in all of chiropractic that relates our original philosophy and intention of adjusting to objective hard evidence.

Chiropractic philosophy and the original science of the profession focused on the understanding that if there is a physical or biomechanical distortion to a vertebra in the spine (called a subluxation), it will result in an alteration to the function of the nerve leaving the spine at that level, and a dysfunction of the organ or extremity that that nerve services.

Dis-ease leading to disease.

This understanding of the body is fundamental in traditional chiropractic literature and practice. Still, it's lost importance in many chiropractic colleges over the last few decades because it causes perpetual strife within the medical associations. Chiropractic colleges have become desperate to be accepted by big brother medicine, so they've started to abandon this fundamental understanding and focus their efforts solely on pain management instead of the body's overall health.

Why would this cause strife within medical associations, you ask?

If chiropractors are concerned with global human health, including organ health and organ function, then we are playing in the same big boy pool as medical doctors and are at risk of taking people off medication and curing diseases. In other words, we are at risk of taking away someone else's paycheck.

The good news is that regardless of the effort to abandon this understanding, the reality cannot be changed just because everyone is trying to turn a blind eye.

If someone walks into my office with pain and numbness in their foot or big toe, they will likely tell me they have sciatica. If it turns out that this is a spinal nerve problem and not a tight muscle in their glute or buttocks (called the piriformis muscle) contracting and pressing on the sciatic nerve, then they would be correct. Most of the time, it is the latter, called *Piriformis Syndrome*, but if it is a true sciatica, then it will be a compression of the spinal nerve leaving the lumbar spine, causing the sciatic pain.

The compression can be the result of either a spinal disc bulge or herniation or compression of the nerve root as it leaves the spine due to a subluxation, acute injury, or degeneration. Regardless of the mechanism, we all understand that this is a very likely and common situation and that when there is compression on the nerve leaving the spine, the sensation and function of the location that the nerve travels to changes. So, if you have a numb, painful, or weak foot, it can be a problem with the spine, not the foot.

But what happens if you have a kidney problem? Or liver disease? Or suffered a heart attack? Or any other condition related to organ function? Could that be related to the spinal nerve being compressed as it leaves the spine from a previous injury? As a matter of fact, it could.

In an effort to disprove the chiropractors in his time, a groundbreaking study was performed by Dr. Henry Windsor, M.D., to evaluate if there was any merit to the grandiose claims being made by chiropractors in the early decades of the profession that they were able to heal individuals of conditions ranging from digestive problems, thyroid dysfunction, heart problems, and even cancer by adjusting their spines and affecting the function of the spinal nerves that service these various diseased organs.

In his 1921 study,[9] Windsor used 50 cadavers from the University of Pennsylvania and 22 feline cadavers, in which he isolated 221 diseased organs. In tracing the innervation of the nerves to these diseased organs from the spine, he found a 95.9% correlation to a minor but noticeable curvature, or displacement in the spine in the segmental area in which the nerve for each diseased organ exited the spine.

In an attempt to disprove chiropractic philosophy, Windsor made one of the greatest contributions to chiropractic science to date and proved the accuracy of the connection between spinal subluxations and organ health —with a 95.9% accuracy rate.

According to this study, a subluxation in the spine at the area where the nerve that feeds a specific organ originates resulted in disease and dysfunction of that organ 95.9% of the time. *This* is what big brother medicine doesn't want you to know and why chiropractic has been public enemy number one to the pharmaceutical giants since its discovery. Interestingly, it was right around this time when the American Medical Association formed its coalition to attack and

---

[9] *Sympathetic Segmental Disturbances: The Evidences of the Association in Dissected Cadavers of Visceral Disease with Vertebral Deformities of the Same Sympathetic Segments#* Medical Times, November 1921, pp. 1-7

defame chiropractic and began the biggest smear campaign in medical history —up until recently.

For the next 60-plus years, the AMA systematically tried to destroy chiropractic by attacking the merit and legitimacy of the profession and the personal reputations of everyone within it. Rumors that chiropractors kill people, cause strokes, paralyze people, and similar claims were perpetuated ad nauseam to the public through fake news articles and fabricated horror stories. Medical schools built into their curriculums systematic disinformation training for new doctors that chiropractors were absolutely, under no circumstances, to be trusted or spoken to. They even went so far as to declare if any medical doctor was found to be associating with a chiropractor, even if they were brother and sister, the medical doctor would lose their license. This continued until 1987 when a chiropractor named Chester A. Wilk, along with ten other co-defendants, sued the AMA. They sued one of the most powerful machines of all time...

And won.

The Wilks case demonstrated that, without question, every rumor and fabricated horror story about chiropractic — many of which you still hear today — are based on false propaganda with no evidence whatsoever to validate the claims. This was a true David vs. Goliath moment in which a marginalized underdog took on the entire American Medical Association and won.

So, where does this leave us today? Well, despite the incredible research that has been conducted throughout the last 125 years validating chiropractic philosophy and the power of an adjustment, along with the countless millions of miracle stories heard and seen around the world in ever chiro office, chiropractic is still being targeted as the medical establishment's primary enemy ¾ only now the attacks are coming both from the outside, as well as from within. Infiltration of chiropractic schools by medically slanted directives has resulted in chiropractors now being trained to work on muscles and provide exercises instead of using the science of chiropractic to heal diseases and change lives. Chiropractic colleges around the world have been tainted with the idea that somehow chiropractic isn't enough and that chiropractors should now aspire instead to be second-rate physiotherapists with an identity crisis.

Though we have grown to be the third largest medical profession world-wide, behind dentistry and allopathic medicine, the chiropractic message and principles of practice have become so watered down and disfigured that many chiropractic practices are almost unrecognizable from the original practices that paved the way for our profession. I can't tell you how many times I have had a new patient in my office who has told me they have been seeing other chiropractors for years but then were completely surprised when I did the first adjustment. When I ask them if they have ever had anything like that done, they reply with something like, "They usually just stretch me out and tape my back," or "he does more muscle release work," or "We spent a lot of time talking about posture, but she never actually touched me." As a profession, we have strayed away from the one thing that we can provide that no one else in the world can ¾ and it's the most valuable thing any chiropractor can do.

So, to all the strong-willed and brave chiropractors out there who know and continue to share the power of the adjustment with their communities, I salute you. And to anyone who is on the edge or nervous about going to one again because they had an unfavorable experience, all I can say is that there are millions of hairstylists out there, and they all cut hair differently. If you get a shitty haircut, you don't decide to never get it cut again; you find a different stylist and get it fixed.

The world is ready for the truth about the human body and who and what we are. People are desperately seeking a specialist who understands the natural processes of the body and who works with them, not against them, to restore and maintain optimal human function in an effort to obtain the highest levels of human health. It's time for us chiropractors to step up and show them what we can do. This is where we can shine, if we can get the message out.

CHAPTER 16

EMOTIONS & ENERGY

Now that we have addressed our physical makeup along with our chemical makeup in previous chapters, let's look again at our energetic makeup. After all, we are energetic bodies, and we require a proper flow of energy to function.

Outside of eating the right foods, how else can we charge our batteries?

It turns out our emotions have a lot to do with it.

Our energetic bodies, just like our physical bodies, are like internal batteries — but these batteries can be charged or drained by forces of an energetic make-up, much in the same way our physical batteries can be affected by our chemical make-up, as discussed previously. Our energetic batteries can be charged through the interaction and absorption of positive energy, and they can be drained through either the interaction with negative energy or by simply expending too much of our energy too frequently.

Love and emotions that stem from the love spectrum, such as gratitude, joy, peace, forgiveness, fulfillment, accomplishment, and all other vibrationally positive emotions, charge our inner battery; while emotions like sadness, grief, guilt, frustration, blame, hate, and all emotions that vibrate with a negative energy work to deplete them.

Think about some of the memories you have that are attached to the experience and feeling of love, for example. When you recall those memories, you tend to feel a literal *warmth* inside, like a comforting blanket or internal hug. You feel warmth in your stomach and warmth in your chest, and your whole being feels cozy and safe. When you feel love or any of the other positive and rejuvenating emotions, your energy increases, you feel happiness, you feel calmness, and you experience comfort permeating through your whole being — like a snuggle wrapping you from the inside out. On top of this, just feeling a positive sensation, that comfort and warmth can also act as a usable electromagnetic charge, resulting in a chemical reaction inside your body. This reaction, and the chemical by-products that result from it, has a direct impact on the turning on and turning off of genetic switches in your DNA that allow you to move from fear into growth and systematically recalibrate your genetic expression to its most optimized state.

Love quite literally changes our DNA expression, and that's a fact. (For more on this, read "The Biology of Belief" by Dr. Bruce Lipton.)

It turns out love has a far larger effect on our physiology than we may have previously considered. Popular expressions, such as "I've got my love to keep me warm" from a famous Christmas song, the universally used "Love is enough," or "Love is the answer," and of course, John Lennon's "Love is all you need" tend to summarize this idea in cute, catchy little phrases that sell lots of products, but what is love, really? Love is, in fact, the *most powerful positive energy in the entire known universe* and the base vibration of the divine.

Love itself is more than a word, an idea, or a passing feeling. Love is a powerful positive energy that permeates through and charges the batteries of the person experiencing it while spreading like an overflowing cup in every direction. Love will fill your batteries and increase your internal energy faster and more effectively than any other force in existence. The true experience of love will fill your core being, your heart, your home, and your entire life in one powerful swoop if you let it.

If you give love and allow love into your life — not just in a romantic way, but in all manners of unconditional love, like loving your neighbor as yourself, loving your enemies as your friends, and loving life as the gift that it is— then that love will fill your life and everything that you are with joy, peace, purpose, and gratitude. Jesus came to the earth to rewrite the laws and left us with one principle that he said to be more important than all the rest: The principle of Love.

Everything is love, and love is everything. That is the true power of love, and that is the essential energy required to adequately charge your internal batteries and renew your true divine energy. Eating and drinking can nourish the body, but they cannot nourish the soul. Food is energy from the outside in; love is energy produced from the inside out. When your soul is filled, your body and life will also be filled. As Jesus said, those who come to me will never thirst (John 4: 13-14). Meaning those who embrace and live in all-encompassing love will never thirst for anything else.

Now, on the other side of this spectrum, emotions such as sadness, frustration, and anger are all sources of energy depletion, and they are sources of soul depletion.

When you feel any of these emotions, you feel hot — your head feels hot, your back feels hot, and your heart races. This is the physiological effect of energy being used and burned off. It is the expelling of energy from your body and the experiential sensation of the energetic draining of your batteries. Guilt, hate, anger, fear, all those things are depletion mechanisms. They take your inner batteries, and they burn them at high rates, depleting them faster than any other mechanism out there, save for intense physical exercise. If love is the essence of all that is good and can rewrite our genetic code for health and optimized expression, then emotions of hate, guilt, anger, and jealousy can do the exact opposite. Studies in epigenetics (Dr. Bruce Lipton – The Biology of Belief) have shown that if you were to fight with someone and then directly afterward take a sample of your DNA, it would have slightly different genetic markers turned on and off than if the DNA was extracted while you were feeling happy, in love, or grateful. These emotions, quite literally, change our DNA and charge or deplete our energetic bodies. So, every change in emotion changes our DNA in some measurable way as an effect.

Let's go a little deeper.

The two polarities of love and fear can be divided further into subcategories of their mechanisms and effects on our bodies.

The first of the negative emotion subcategories is the subcategory of anger and fear. These two emotions are strong, powerful emotions that expel energy from your body at a high rate, emitting it out into the world in a process similar to combustion. When a log or fire burns, there is a dense, internally stored energy that quietly exists and quietly maintains its shape in the material world through a dense structure and the condensed, stored energy. However, when an alternate source of energy is introduced that is enough to create a combustion reaction to that material, then there is a spontaneous emittance of high levels of energy as it is freed from the material state it was in. The energy that was stored inside of the material holding it in space is deconstructed and combusted to release its energy back out into the air, leading to the destruction of the fabric of the material in which it was housed and the liberation of the energy back into the source.

Fear and anger have the same effects on the human body. Fear and anger are both very fast, quick sources of combustion in which our internal structures are converted to heat and released back to the source in the process of internal combustion. During the experience of these emotions, not only is a large amount of energy being emitted and lost but that energy mingles with negative emotions and negative frequencies as it is sent back out to the world. Our internal reaction creates a domino effect, and the energy we give off spreads the emotions we experience to others around us. Just like joy is contagious, so is fear and anger.

The other remaining negative emotions, such as guilt, sadness, regret, shame, and jealousy, are also effective in reducing our own internal batteries — but in a slightly different way.

Instead, these emotions drain our internal energy in a way that would more appropriately fit the analogy of leaving a light on the inside of a vehicle overnight. This light, though it may be less noticeable than your engine being on fire, will still draw constant energy from the battery of the vehicle, and over some time, it will deplete the entirety of the stored energy. This small drainage, over a long period, adds up to be enough to drain the battery and cause an incredible amount of frustration. Again, these emotions have the same effect on the body. They slowly but consistently draw energy from your internal batteries and your internal energy sources, resulting in a gradual but obvious depletion of your internal energy over time. This slow but steady depletion results in a decline in happiness, a reduction in the feelings and sensations of love, and a loss of hope and motivation as your energy falls lower and lower every day. Like a constant, nagging voice in the background, these emotions rob you of moments of true and uninhibited happiness by sucking away your internal life force.

The presence of one or more of these energetic vampires in a person's life inevitably leads to people looking for ways to compensate for these emotions, usually turning to easy and quick dopamine dumps to use extreme highs to fight the constant lows. It is no coincidence that these emotions are often linked to illness and chronic disease. If your body is always running on an energetic deficit, it will inevitably begin to decay. We find that when there is a long-term depletion of energy in someone's life, it is often linked to one or more specific negative events. So, the emotions of guilt, sadness, and regret in our bodies do not just float around randomly in space with nothing attached to them. These emotions are fixated on events, which become stored in our electromagnetic bodies, also called our auric bodies. These auric bodies are intrinsically linked with the physical body. Often, these negative emotions become intertwined both in the physical tissues that were involved in the negative experience, like scar tissue from an injury, as well as the electromagnetic body that holds this event in our holographic blueprint.

When we discussed our biofield earlier in the book and provided evidence showing portions of our biofield having decreased signal or tangled signal from some traumatic event, this pattern goes hand in hand with these negative emotions. In fact, often it is these emotions that create the distortions in the field. When there is guilt or sadness attached to events in our life, whether they be a small event or a large one, if these events are not cleared from the body and these emotions are not dealt with appropriately, they become small tangles within our energetic and emotional bodies that can continue to cause problems, even if the physical injuries of an event are being treated. For a good visual, think of these tangles as black holes constantly sucking our energy from our physical and energetic bodies by creating a flaw in the hologram. When energy is being drawn into these black holes, it is being robbed from places that need this electromagnetic energy to function properly. These tangles steal energy from us and restrict the flow of life force to certain areas of the body, eventually leading to disease.

Particular organs are responsible for housing particular emotions. The long-term effect of these negative emotions leads to disease in areas of the body where these emotions are attached to and stored, along with disease in areas of the body in which the physical or emotional blockage has limited the flow of life force. This is the fundamental basis of chiropractic philosophy: thoughts, traumas, and toxins can create energetic and physical blockages that limit life force energy, which, over time, will first result in dis-ease of a given area or organ and eventually lead to the formal development of disease if not corrected.

Now, going back to the variety of negative emotions, though they affect our bodies in slightly different ways, fear and anger can also cause problems with health and lead to dis-ease; however, these emotions result in different types of health problems. These emotions, when left long enough to manifest dis-ease in the body, will lead to conditions of disease such as heart disease, liver disease, increased opportunistic infections, and illnesses surrounding decreased immune system function.

Fear and anger reduce our immune system way that is different from slow-acting negative emotions because they deplete our energy in very fast, combustible, and dramatic ways. That energy expelled is taken from the energy required for a functioning? appropriate immune system function. So, while sadness and guilt are slow-acting emotions that result in long-term depletion, fear and anger are fast-acting emotions that result in higher-level depletion in a short period. Along with the depletion of energy, fear and anger also destroy cells as a result of the forces of this combustion, which also have a direct effect on our internal organs and biomes. Given that these are quick-combustion emotions, they are usually shorter-lived, which is the reason they are not as closely linked with long-term diseases; however, as stated above, if allowed to exist within a person unchecked for longer periods, they can result in heart and liver problems, since these are the organs typically associated with the processing of these two emotions.

Since fear and anger are the quickest acting and most combustible of all emotions, meaning they are the fastest to provoke and release the most amount of energy out into the world, they are very useful for collecting and permeating a high frequency of energy across the world. When the world is in fear, energy is being combusted and released into the atmosphere at incredibly high rates. This free energy could be used and harvested if one had the technology or knowledge of how to do so; however, for the average person, the experience of this can still be palpable.

I am sure you have had an experience of walking into a room and instantly feeling the energy is off and unsettled. There is a high amount of energy being released from every person who is experiencing anger or fear; hence, when there is news about something bad or scary in the world, the energy of fear is tangible in the air all around you. Energy is a very strong force that permeates our world and is the main driving force of current media and entertainment sectors. Touching back on the previous chapters about subtle energy and signals passing through us and having a direct effect on our physiology, what effects do you think strong energies of fear and anger coursing through the ether would have on a person who was to walk within their pathway? Remember going out into public over the last three years? Was it an enjoyable experience?

If you are anything like me, who is quite sensitive to these subtle signals, the answer would be a big, giant HELL NO!

On the positive side, however, despite these forces being incredibly strong, powerful, and easy to ignite in people, they are not nearly as powerful as the *power of love, compassion, and connection.* Think about Star Wars — the dark side of the force was easier to tap into, but it was no match for someone who mastered the force of the light side. Emotions related to love are incredibly engulfing and cleansing; however, we can't deny the fact that these emotions are quite elusive in our current world — especially compared to fear and anger. After all, we don't have multi-million-dollar news networks dedicated to making us feel safe and happy like we do the ones dedicated to driving fear and division.

The truth is that love is a frequency of energy that is systematically and purposefully trained out of us. Love leads to connection, and it is extremely uniting and powerful. For that exact reason, those who currently have power of any kind do not want us to feel loved or connected. That could lead to dangerous levels of cooperation, and the key to keeping power is to limit any form of cooperation between the people below you.

Black or white.

Gay or straight.

Red or blue.

Vaccinated or unvaccinated.

Divide and conquer.

Doom and despair.

To show the power of this indoctrination of aversion to love, think of when you hear somebody say, "Everything is love," or "I love you," or "Love thy neighbor." Unless coming from a person you love romantically, all these phrases tend to elicit a negative knee-jerk internal reaction in an individual who hears them. They sound cliche, cheesy, or corny, and certainly not powerful or healing.

This aversion has made it so that instead of love being a word that carries energy that should instantly elevate our internal beings and attune us to a higher frequency when we hear it, love is instead a word that carries energy that we have been *conditioned* to turn away from, block, and react negatively to at just the *mention* of it.

Something that any individual who spends enough time researching and reading into the big questions of reality and studying topics such as the frequencies of life, unaltered alternative health care, esoteric science and wisdom, noetic sciences, religion, and current theoretical physics will eventually be forced to realize is, *love is everything.*

It's not cliché, and it's not just silly-sounding hyperbole. Love is all, and love is the great tuning frequency that can extinguish fear, anger, hate, and all other negative emotions. As soon as we tune our energetic and emotional bodies to love, everything in our life changes.

Love is all, and it changes all.

Love is like the energy of the sun, which splits through the clouds on a stormy day and illuminates everything. When that ray illuminates your inner being, you instantly become better in every possible way. The light shines on all areas of your life, and the darkness is chased away. This is the power of love from within our internal energetic beings to illuminate our lives in a new light and instantaneously transform the world around and within us.

In the same way that the sun is the main charging factor for all life forms on this planet, love is the main charging factor for humans. Without love, we are constantly and hopelessly trying to plug our batteries into short-term energy through dopamine bursts as our internal batteries are depleted at faster and faster rates. We are constantly looking at the low battery signal flashing and desperately searching for new energy sources, knowing full well our devices will soon shut off unless we find something new to fill them.

This emergency state in which we continuously find ourselves is a state of panic and survival, purposefully crafted to keep us weak and distracted. To merely survive is to merely scramble to plug your phone in right before it dies and then take it out as soon as the low battery signal turns off, over and over ad infinitum. When you find that short-term energy source, you have a short period of minor relief. Still, the panic never fully subsides because you know that that low battery signal is coming back any minute, and when it does, you better get to a charger fast, so you rush from place to place, always keeping in the front of your mind how close you are to falling apart. It's almost like a game of musical chairs — when the music is on, you walk around the chair, but you never let yourself get too far or think about anything too distant and distracting because you know at any moment the music can shut off and you will need to sit down.

Fast.

Only in this situation it's not just a game; our lives are at stake. Our health, our families, our marriages, our careers, our reputations.

Our futures.

This is how most people live their lives, running from one dopamine dump to another, ignoring what is much more important in the world while looking for quick bursts of energy to sustain them as they frantically search for a more reliable and long-term source. Though these spikes fill them up and satisfy them quickly, the satisfaction drops even faster, and they are left exactly where they were before, or worse. Think of these dopamine dumps like cooking in a microwave. When you heat something in a microwave, it gets hot fast — very, very fast; however, when you pull it out and leave it on the counter for a moment, you will notice that even though it reached the same peak temperature as cooking on a stove, the middle still may be cold. The whole piece of food cools off extremely fast. This is because the actual mechanisms of heating inside a microwave are completely different from the mechanisms of heating on a stove or in an oven. The microwave provides a quick, convenient response; however, the food is never cooked evenly, and the effect is not long-lasting. Not to mention that the effects of heating food via the microwave are harmful to human health, just like using dopamine as your main energy source would be.

At the risk of sounding redundant, another analogy would be maintaining a fire with small amounts of kindling versus large logs— the kindle will burn up quickly and require constant restocking. In contrast, the large logs will maintain the fire much longer and with much less tending required. Yes, sometimes a fire requires kindling to start, but to sustain it long-term, large logs are mandatory unless you want to feed in a new handful of kindling every few minutes.

This analogy allows us to turn to the underlying reason why dopamine is a poor long-term fuel — and it's based on neurology.

Kindling versus large logs represents the difference between dopamine and serotonin, which are both neurotransmitters in the brain. Serotonin is the molecule of comfort, and, along with oxytocin, these molecules work as the chemical signals for love, security, and long-term happiness, while dopamine is the molecule and chemical signal of pleasure. Going back to the cooking analogy, when we cook on the stove, we slowly and evenly heat something — much slower than the microwave. However, once it is hot, it *stays hot* for a lot longer. Using the stove, we have slowly increased the energy within all the molecules of that food appropriately and sustainably, which results in natural and complete cooking without damaging the integrity of proteins inside the food. Once we remove this food from the heat, that heat is stored within those cells for a longer time because all the cells have raised their internal vibration while having the time to adapt their protein structures to resonate with the physical changes of the heat. When we cook in a microwave, by comparison, we induce a large-scale wave of high-level energy that affects the water molecules at a much different rate than food molecules. So, the high-level energy heats the water molecules, but it does not heat the structural molecules of the food at the same rate. This results in a massive spike in energy to the borders of the food as the water heats quickly, but the proteins in the food do not. Because the resonance of every other molecule of that food is not at the same resonance as the affected water molecules, the water molecules cause damage and degradation of the protein structures of the food, then evaporate and release from that food. As soon as it's taken out of the microwave, the molecules of water quickly evaporate and cool, while the molecules of the food become permanently altered by the intense transition of heat.

Ok, now bear with me.

All this food and fire talk is relevant to the human body in that dopamine can be like both the *kindling and the microwave* in which you can get a quick and immediate response, but it is not only *unsustainable*; it can also be *harmful*.

As our dopamine receptors continue to be abused inside of our brains, they actually begin to be less sensitive to the input — meaning they require more dopamine to get the same effects over time. This is very much like putting a fire together using only kindling, but once the fire actually starts to heat up, trying to maintain a fire with kindling is impossible as the heat of the fire rises higher and higher. In the beginning, each piece of kindling lasted a few minutes, but as the fire temperature rises, each piece now only lasts about 30-45 seconds. Each piece of kindling will be burnt almost immediately; there is no lasting energy inside of that kindling to allow for a long-term, sustained fire. More dopamine is required, meaning more thrill and pleasure are needed to satisfy those receptors as they become less and less sensitive.

This is where serotonin comes in for the win. Serotonin is the big log you can lay down that will burn for hours.

This slow desensitization of receptor sites is why we have to start consciously feeding our brains with molecules that actually elicit long-term happiness instead of short-term pleasure. We must seek happiness through calmness and love, not through pleasure.

Gratitude and service, not impulse and consumption.

Depending on your level of interest in esoteric sciences, this idea may seem self-evident, or it may seem completely new. Either way, let's take a look at the evidence we can find for it within our historical records.

THE TRUE MESSAGE OF ALL RELIGIONS

All religions and ancient philosophies speak of different methods of the attainment of peace through enlightenment or salvation; however, if you collectively look at them all and remove the specific names and finer details that are argued over that set them apart, boiled down to their base principles what you are left with are instructions for how to rid yourself of negative emotions that deplete your internal batteries and a guide to increase your internal energy by service to others, and the unchanging principle of love.

When we're happy — and I mean truly happy — we have a sense of security and comfort. It's much like the feeling when you first lay down in bed after a long day. The sheets are so cool and soft, and the duvet gets wrapped around you perfectly like a cloud. Or like the feeling of a warm blanket embracing you while sitting in front of a fireplace on a cold winter's day, or seeing the smile of someone you love, or coming home to your loving family after a long, hard day and knowing that everyone there loves you and is happy to see you.

All these experiences result in the experience of love and result in serotonin and oxytocin being released inside our body, like putting a big, giant log onto the fire. The warmth you feel inside during each one of these experiences is not just metaphorical — it's actually a physical energy that fills every part of your being, which allows you to sit back and relax, knowing you can just let it burn. You feel secure knowing that you are full and do not need to constantly add new logs to the fire or run to find the next closest charger. You no longer need new dopamine dumps every five minutes because the love you feel is more than enough and fills all your reserves. It is enough to last you a long, long time. Even a lifetime.

Like the soldiers who fought in the worst conditions imaginable in WWII who persevered by constantly looking at the single photo of their wives they carried with them in their pockets. That was enough to get them through and, for many, to get them back home. Without love, we are always trying to fill a cup with a hole in the bottom; with love, that cup is filled to the brim, and we stop looking for anything else to pour into it.

FALSE SUBSTITUTES FOR LOVE:
Dopamine and Mechanisms of Addiction

Depletion of dopamine receptor sensitivity, as outlined above, does more than just keep us in search of the next bump; it is the foundation of all forms of addiction. Whether it's an addiction to drugs, food, pornography, or social media and the constant need for validation, these are all forms of a dopamine-dependent response, and all result in and are maintained by, dopamine-directed desensitization of those neuroreceptors in our brains.

In our current society, we tend to look at addiction treatment in ways that are very largely ineffective. The reason for this is that we attempt to remove the sources of dopamine dumps without looking for ways to continue the fire burning without the kindling. We take away the kindling and extinguish the fire instead of providing logs.

Let's face it: it is very difficult for most people to break free from an addiction, and those that have usually end up replacing it with something else that is also addiction-forming but hopefully healthier in the long run. This is because there is not enough emphasis placed on habits and actions that *sustain internal feelings of satiation and contentment*, i.e., serotonin and oxytocin-producing actions. Or, quite basically, sources of genuine love.

So if you want to keep a fire going but don't want to put kindling in every three seconds, you need to put in larger logs that have a bigger form of energy that gives you enough time that you can sit down and actually enjoy the fire you've created with the people you love, and allow yourself to rest for long enough to feel content. This is the neuro-chemical dynamics of addiction, but it is also the base neurochemical dynamics that underpin the entirety of our internal mental health. As mental health affects our physical health, these neurodynamics have a huge impact on our internal health and well-being as well.

Physical health is based on the same principles as mental health and addiction. Physical health comes from a high state of internal energy with low levels of energetic disruption or blockages anywhere within the physical body and the bioelectric field around us.

For physical health to be restored and maintained, energy must be at a high enough level inside of our bodies and be able to flow back and forth through all levels and systems of our physical anatomy as well as our energetic anatomy, with ease, abundance, and without restriction. When this is the case, the result is high levels of health and joy in life. When this is not the case, we experience discomfort and dis-ease, which can result in physical and mental disease states. It is important that this principle is understood because it is the underlying constant of all other things written about in this book. Without high levels of internally produced energy that is free of disruption and blockages, we cannot set up appropriately functioning and responding mental, physical, or energetic bodies. We cannot properly discuss cycles and transitions in the human body based on environmental stimuli without an appropriately calibrated and functional internal environment to allow for those signals to be properly interpreted and the actions of our body to be appropriately carried out. Without this fundamental base being present in an individual, everything else is subject to error and inappropriate responses to the messages of both internal and external signals. Essentially, without a properly balanced and uninhibited nervous system and control center, all other signals and cycles will be interpreted and responded to incorrectly, and dis-ease will be inevitable.

Striving for and maintaining a balanced and calibrated union of our mental, physical, emotional, and spiritual bodies will result in a properly functioning and healthy individual. This balance will also allow us to interact with signals presented to us from both within and without the body in accurate and appropriate ways, creating not only a truly healthy human being but also a highly adaptable and integrated member of any environment or situation we may find ourselves in.

CHAPTER 17

CREATION VS. CONSUMPTION

"If you bring forth what is within you, what you bring forth will save you. If you do not bring forth what is within you, what you do not bring forth with destroy you". – Jesus, The Gospel of Thomas

In nature, nothing can stay in perfect inertia, so at all times, things are either being created or destroyed.

The physics principle of inertia states that something will stay exactly how it is or stay in the motion and trajectory it is going until an opposing force alters it. If all forces on an object are equal, then that object will not move, but if there is any imbalance in the forces, the stronger one and the magnitude of difference will dictate how fast an object will move and in what direction. This is Newton's First Law of Motion.

In our organic bodies and material world, destructive forces surround us at all times. Forces such as gravity, weak and strong electromagnetic forces, friction, and radioactive decay represent forces that constantly act upon all matter at all times, thus preventing a true perpetual state of inertia from existing in the natural world. Therefore, Newton's laws suggest an idea that, in true reality, isn't quite possible. It plays out very similarly to Plato's theory of forms mentioned earlier.

To maintain any material thing and any living organism in existence, the innate force of creation is in a constant battle with the material forces of destruction. Innate intelligence, according to the major premise of chiropractic, is what maintains all matter in existence and constantly gives to it all its properties, thus maintaining it in existence. This is also known as the First Principle of Chiropractic. Innate builds. Natural decay, also known as entropy, destroys.

To perform the duty of creation, innate forces and intelligence require certain fuels and resources to actively and effectively carry out the blueprint of creation from idea to material reality. These resources are the energetic currencies living organisms use as building blocks to bring the blueprint of life into existence.

The first Law of Thermodynamics is the Law of Conservation of Energy, which states that energy can neither be created nor destroyed, only converted. As such, all living organisms cannot create or destroy energy; rather, they convert the energy of sunlight, food, and electromagnetic potential into material bodies using the guiding force of innate intelligence coupled with conscious will.

This is the law and process of the material world down to the basic building blocks of life and the mystery of life on a simple production-destruction level. However, it is a highly simplified version of the material recycling process all matter in existence undertakes since it does not account for or address the subtle forces on matter that we cannot yet comprehend.

Regardless of what the egomaniacs of the world want you to believe, there is still much mystery in life and much we do not yet know. The human body and human experience are about as fully explored as the ocean — meaning we really haven't even scratched the surface — but despite the simplification, the above principle remains true.

It also remains true on another level of our reality that we likely experience and interact with on a much more regular basis — at least on a conscious level, that is, the social level.

As the wisdom of Hermes Trismegistus states famously in his Principle of Correspondence: "As above, so below."

All processes and patterns repeat no matter how big or how small you scale them. Creation and destruction are the two opposing poles in balance in all aspects of the physical and material world. The only way to escape this cycle is to become a completely energetic being — aka a divine soul — because, remember, energy cannot be created or destroyed. Therefore, energy and the soul must live on.

SOCIAL IMPLICATIONS

Just as creation and consumption are the two opposing poles of the same frequency in cellular and biological life, they are also two opposing poles of the same energy frequency in our social and cultural lives.

I believe we are all born naturally creative. I believe it is not only our natural innate state to be creative but that *it is our duty on a soul level to create.*

Every individual on this planet will have a unique experience of life. If you take a single situation in which 100 people are involved, there will be 100 different experiences of the situation. We are all unique beings, and we exist as unique entities that have come to this earth to have unique experiences. Even if the same soul were to incarnate 1,000 times, assuming reincarnation is possible, it would have 1,000 unique experiences, which is the whole point. We are here to *experience* — but we are also here to *create.*

It is also our soul's duty to *create based on our gifts and our experience* to *share* our experiences, emotions, and unique abilities with the other souls on this planet, ultimately contributing to the collective experience that can be tapped into by all living beings culminating in the library of shared human experience over time. Think about how one single artist can create a song that allows millions to experience something deeply personal and intimate just by hearing it. All different experiences, all from the same catalyst. This, I believe, is our duty. Every one of us, in our unique ways, contributes our own catalysts for others to use to have their own unique experiences.

But how many of us are living up to this duty? How many of us are truly creating as much as we can or being conscious of what we are creating? And even if we are creating, how many of us are sharing it?

Take yourself for example. I can almost guarantee that there is something you have been thinking and dreaming about creating for a long time but have not yet found the time or motivation to do it. Or the guts to share it.

Even more likely, you have started but not finished it.

Well, here is my advice: *Do it.*

Do it Now.

Don't worry about it being perfect; just bring your vision to life and let it take shape. We need it, and nobody ever in the world, no matter how many more years of this earth or people that come into existence, will ever, ever, *ever* create what you are thinking of creating, not exactly how you will.

Either you do it, or no one will.

No one will ever make your exact creation *except you*. Even if I were to write this chapter tomorrow instead of today, it would not be the same chapter. It would be written with slightly different words. Different punctuation. Different style. *Because that would be the expression of my directed consciousness at that period, instead of this one,* creation is the stroke of genius that comes from the divine playing through you as an agent of expression. It is a gift from God. But with the stroke of genius and the flash of inspiration, the human contribution is the *work*. It's the time and the tenacity to finish the project and bring it to life.

The divine is doing its job; now we have to do ours.

THE CONSEQUENCES OF *NOT* CREATING

So, with this many souls in the world who are not creating what they are destined and energetically called to create, what happens with all this unused creative energy? It cannot just be destroyed, so instead, it gets turned from potential energy for creation into energy used for consumption.

From creation to consumption and from fulfillment into frustration. This may seem like an inert transition, but changing the expression of this divine energy of creativity from creation to consumption affects not just your mood and sense of fulfillment but the whole world and our society's function. It is purposefully harnessed by corporations and the whole reason we are in the place we are in as a society today.

It also has a dramatic effect on your health and relationships as well. Why do you think corporations would rather a large majority of people consume instead of creating? Well, I'm sure it's pretty obvious.

BUY, BUY, *BUY*

We have become a world and society based on obsessive and addictive levels of overconsumption. In every possible way. Even during a worldwide pandemic in which any rational human should be saving and penny-pinching, what are we all doing? Buying, buying, buying, buying.

Non. Stop.

Hold, please; the Amazon driver is at my door.

We are amid the supposed greatest worldwide pandemic that has ever occurred, barreling towards a pre-planned and incredibly obvious economic crash and resource shortage … yet we can't stop buying shit we don't need. Why? Because our collective global creativity has not only been stifled, our *freedom to even have our own individual thoughts and insights has been stolen from us.*

We are currently living in the most suffocating and controlling state that anyone in our lifetimes has ever experienced in the realm of creative expression. So, in a culture built on exploiting and creating consumption addiction, when a crisis hits and creative outlets are taken away, we move towards our pre-trained coping outlets, and search for dopamine dumps in Amazon checkout pages and FedEx delivery drivers. We are attempting to fill our empty internal reservoirs that are typically filled with even minor amounts of creative energy with a substitution of massive amounts of consumption energy.

The result?

Frustration. Sorrow. Depression — ever-reducing times that dopamine spikes satisfy us, and ever-increasing attempts to find more through the avenue of consumption and instant gratification.

But we won't, because we can't.

Consumption is the equivalent of destruction. It's the *use* of our resources instead of harnessing the *creation* of our resources. We can never fill our reserves by destruction. We can never grow a tree by eating its fruit. We have to plant a seed.

Creation is planting the tree and growing our resources.

We must create.

We must allow ourselves permission to break these mental chains and invite ourselves to experience the thrill and satisfaction of our own original thoughts, ideas, and creative expressions once again. We must allow ourselves permission to entertain all novel ideas that come our way because *that is exactly how we grow and how we will personally and collectively get out of this mess! Not just the mess of the last three years but the mess of the downward spiral of the human condition.*

We cannot allow ourselves to go on any longer, accepting that what we are allowed to think or say can be dictated by someone else — some distant theoretical authority. We are creative beings, and we must embrace our differences and create! Diversity is, and always has been, essential in the resilience of any group, lifeform, or thing.

Nobody enjoys anything generic.

We are not designed to see the world the same as our neighbor. We are not designed to all have the same homogenous thoughts and agree on all the important ideas and topics. If this were the case, we would have never heard of Biggie Smalls, Elvis, or Nirvana. Einstein would have been a shoemaker. We would have never heard the speech of Martin Luther King Jr. We would never have switched from horses to cars. And if this were the case, there would be *absolutely no advancement of our civilization or species. Ever.*

In fact, it would mean that there would be no advancement of *any species* ever. Or any *thing* ever!

There couldn't be.

Darwinian evolution is predicated on our differences, creating divergence in traits and qualities, leading to different levels of survival for certain groups of each species in certain environments. If we do not allow original thought, which leads to novel ideas and actions, then we will cease the advancement of our species and set ourselves up for extinction. The world is always changing, so if we stop, then we can no longer be compatible with the world.

If a species has diverging actions, which lead to diverging qualities and traits, then in all environments and situations, one of those divergent variations will, by absolute necessity of fact, have an advantage over the other. There can be no other way.

Regardless of how large or how small that advantage/disadvantage discrepancy is, there must, by absolute fact, be one. Over time, these diverging qualities may evolve, expand, and create a larger difference and larger advantage/disadvantage discrepancy.

Now, do you know what the innate purpose of this could be?

It means that if an event happens that challenges the very survival of a species, the more variation within that species and the more variation of traits, the higher the likelihood that at least one of those groups will survive to continue the species. The more variation in a species, the more variety of challenging events can be survived.

Do you see? It is not only our responsibility and natural innate duty to create and diversify; it is actually the smartest thing we could do as a species to guarantee our survival in the face of any threat. And it is the *only* way to continue to progress and evolve as a species in any way.

CREATION FACILITATES HEALTH

Creative energy is a very powerful energy that exists inside all of us. When not actively used and discharged through creative endeavors, it builds inside our physical bodies and becomes toxic. It transmutes negatively from a positive energy to one that is damaging to us.

Simply put, unexpressed creative energy remains in the body as frustration, regret, and negative self-worth, which leads to the *creation* of disease.

Nature always finds a way to use potential energy, so if you won't consciously use the energy to create, then the energy will find a way to create in a different way.

As stated previously, the opposite of creation is consumption. Consumption equals destruction. That energy, if not used and expelled inside yourself, stays and becomes energy that creates illness by converting to the destruction of your physical, mental, emotional, and energetic bodies.

Not only does the body keep score (great book, by the way, by Dr. Bessel Van Der Kolk) of all the physical and emotional events in your life, it remembers all the areas in which your divine spark and divine energy had the potential to be expressed but was not.

All those potential outcomes are stored in your energetic, emotional, and physical bodies.

All the possibilities of your creation already exist somewhere in the ether, and they are being projected onto you for a reason. It is your responsibility, even your duty, and the best thing you can do for your health, to channel that energy and bring the energetic blueprint into real physical manifestation in this dimension. You would not be sent the signals and not be receiving the divine inspiration if you weren't supposed to act on it.

You are being called to create. It's what makes you special — because your creation will be special.

Through your existence and all the choices, actions, and words you express throughout your life, along with all the works of art and conscious expressions you experience and create, you will write your own story and create your ripple that will continue far longer and far further than you could ever imagine. You create your legacy.

You are here to create. You are here to share who and what you are, and how you experience the world through pieces of unique creation. Unique creations result in unique inspirations in others. Even if you never share them with anyone, bringing them into the physical world is an act of transmutation from the mental to the physical plane. It will raise your confidence level and help you train your mind and body to know that creation is exactly what you are designed to do. Then maybe, after enough time, you will share what you have created with the rest of us.

So go create.

The world needs it more than you know.

* * *

The next portion of this book is based on my own creations and unique ideas. These are ideas that have come to me through my own divine sparks of inspiration and made their way to these pages to share with you. I hope you enjoy, and perhaps even agree with, the theories I am about to present, because I believe they could rewrite how we see the role and function of the human immune system and our body's innate healing properties.

PART II

NEW IDEAS TO CONSIDER

CHAPTER 18

SOMETHING OLD, SOMETHING NEW

Up to this point in the book, everything I have written has been based on someone else's work and ideas. Tested and true. As with most medical and health-based books, the one writing the information is merely the individual delivering the knowledge they had spent years researching and discovering. It is important to have individuals who take on this role because the power of information is only achieved when it is interpreted and understood properly and then communicated succinctly to spread that understanding.

Going forward in these chapters, my role will change from a simple communicator of someone else's ideas to a communicator of my own. In the upcoming chapters, I will present my very own original ideas about the human body and proper human function that complement the understandings already laid out. These theories have been cultivated and groomed over the last five years and have been developed through the synthesis of ideas from all the information I have researched and learned both in my formal education as well as in my parallel curriculum of personal study. Though the ideas may seem profound to some or very basic to others, I suggest that regardless of the initial feelings about them, they will play a pivotal role in reframing the way we see the human body and human health as a whole. As you will see, the true function and natural processes we go through as we progress through the year have been colored and distorted by the interests of pharmaceutical companies. Essentially, natural processes have become symptoms of illness, and basic laws of the body have been ignored and disregarded.

Despite these being original ideas in their formation, I wish to say that though I have done extensive research into these realms of study for many years, it would be impossible to know absolutely all the research and resources related to these topics worldwide. That being said, I wish to acknowledge that if someone somewhere held any of these ideas previously, then I would like to commend them for their work and have no need to claim ownership if that is the case, but to the best of my knowledge, these ideas, as they are presented, in the way they are presented, are my own.

SEASONAL SLOUGHING/ CONTINUOUS BACTERIAL PRIMING THEORY

There's a process that I would like to talk about now that, to the best of my knowledge, is not a currently known or previously discussed theory regarding the human immune response to changes in seasonal cycles, but one that we all experience on a bi-yearly, and sometimes seasonal basis. Over the last few years, this new and emerging theory has slowly become clear to me as I have observed its effect on myself and those around me. I hope to open the door to its discussion and verification upon the publication of this text, openly asking for scientists and researchers to begin the process of validating (or disproving) these claims. What I am choosing to call this emerging theory is Seasonal Sloughing Theory, or Seasonal Bacterial Priming, as part of a greater, more universal principle of Continuous Bacterial Priming Theory.

Seasonal Sloughing and Continuous Bacterial Priming take place inside the bodies of every human, and potentially some animals, on a seasonal basis or when exposed to a new climate or environment. The process is much like the one we see in many other places in nature. All things in nature respond to seasons and cycles, such as environmental changes, and humans are no different.

We have known and observed the response to these cycles in many other organisms in nature, from trees, flowers, fungi, rabbits, butterflies, and even snakes. The debate on how we develop the human immune system has been a well-publicized ongoing battle between two main existing theories of disease, namely the Germ theory (spearheaded by Pasteur) and the Terrain Theory, originally traced back to the work of Bechamp. (It is possible that Pasteur plagiarized Beauchamp's work and altered it to fit his model, based on the research done by author Ethal Douglas Hume in her book *Bechamp or Pasteur? A Lost Chapter in the History of Biology*)

All natural organisms have cycles they move through. Often, these cycles have some relation to the seasons and the changes in the seasonal environments. We have trees that transition every year from green, lush leaves in the spring and summer to beautiful colors in the fall, then proceed to undergo a form of suicide of these beautiful leaves, resulting in shedding, leaving the branches empty throughout winter, only to restart the cycle in spring. As the seasons begin to change from summer to winter, a rabbit's coat changes from brown to white in an evolutionary effort to better camouflage against the changing environment. Snakes are constantly shedding skin as they grow throughout the year. Butterflies and caterpillars somehow morph into a different version of themselves based on their internal clocks that signal to them it is time to make this drastic and complete transformation. Bears eat constantly throughout the warm months to put on the fat needed to survive winter, then climb inside a cave and fall asleep for three to five months.

We see these phenomena all over the planet and in almost all animal kingdoms and intuitively understand these transitions are fundamental and innate to almost every organism in nature; however, it seems like we have turned a blind eye and missed the fact that these timely and predictable transitions may occur in humans as well.

The premise of Seasonal Sloughing Theory is that humans respond to subtle signals in the environment in a similar way other plants and animals do, and we use these signals to initiate a recalibration of our internal environments to better suit upcoming external environments. We respond to subtle signals in changing weather and climate conditions, which trigger a physical response that allows us not only to survive but thrive in the new season, or any new environment we're introduced to. I believe that our internal bacterial environments are designed to recalibrate to best survive the current climate, and the biome is altered to accommodate the demands of the upcoming season year-round. These recalibrations result in many forms of expulsion mechanisms that are innately built into our bodily functions, which have been mistaken over human scientific development to be symptoms of illness.

This idea provides a different explanation for the predictability of the seasonal cold and flu and flies in the face of the currently understood mechanisms of the cold and flu symptomatology.

Existing germ theory models used to explain the seasonal cold and flu say that our immune systems decrease in strength at these predictable times because of changes in vitamin D and yearly mutations to cold and flu bugs and viruses. That, just like a movie premiering on a set date, these new variants and mutations present themselves at the same time of year, every single year, and their appearance coincides with the times our immune system predictably weakens due to changes in sun exposure. According to current paradigms, every year, we are exposed to new opportunistic bacteria and viruses that float around in the air, which results in them invading our bodies due to their new mutations, which allow them to pass our immune system that only has antibodies to fight off the previous variants. It's easier for bacteria to penetrate our systems when our immune systems are compromised from lowered vitamin D levels, so this is the predictable time to get sick. Then, the body's immune response kicks in every year to fight off these newly mutated invaders. If it is successful, we'll live another season with new immunity to that particular new variant exclusively, along with all old ones — only to do it all over again the next season.

I do not believe this theory to be entirely incorrect, but I believe it is flawed. I still believe we can be exposed to bacteria and viruses that can create an immune response, such as being exposed to contaminated meat that causes flu-like symptoms as you experience food poisoning and expel the dangerous contaminants; however, I believe it to be flawed in claiming that all cold and flu symptoms experienced yearly are a result of this and that there is nothing we can do to protect ourselves except take some yearly shot and hope that the god-like minds of the pharmaceutical companies perfected this year's concoction to save us from our wholly inadequate bodies. *It also completely misses the more logical process of the body's natural bacterial cycling process*, which I am presenting here.

Instead of this endless cycle of our bodies battling with new and ever-changing mutations of bacteria and viruses whose sole purpose is to kill us, I would like to put forward the idea that in response to seasonal changes, our bodies perform an innate evolutionary function of burning off, expelling, and altogether sloughing off the bacteria from inside our systems that were required to effectively adapt us to the previous environment but are no longer ideal for the upcoming environment. This allows us to recalibrate our internal environment to protect us more efficiently from the upcoming new external environment. In this manner, symptoms of the seasonal cold and flu are just innate sloughing mechanisms designed to clear the elements of the no longer-suited biome and begin the reconstruction of a new biome that is more appropriate for the upcoming environment.

Just like trees, humans shed our bacterial leaves only to have them replaced by new, more appropriate ones for the upcoming season or the new novel environment in which we have found ourselves. This would explain why there is a spring, fall, and winter version of the cold and flu season. Seasonal sloughing has to take place in all three of these seasons (potentially four seasons if you live somewhere with a fairly drastic distinction between spring and summer) to adapt to the new climate, as well as the more general continuous bacteria priming when we are introduced to a new environment with novel climate stimuli and bacterial ecosystem, such as when we travel.

It's worth noting that this is written in my living room in Canada on a winter day while it is -27 degrees Celsius. The effects of these seasonal changes may not be as drastic or prominent in areas of the world that do not have as drastic changes in seasons, as the purpose of this innate mechanism is to adapt us to a change in the environment adequately. If the environment remains consistent year-round, say somewhere like Hawaii, then the observation of these transitions may be negligible or almost nonexistent.

As stated above in the compare and contrast, I believe the view held and perpetuated by the mainstream regarding seasonal colds and flu symptoms is erroneous. As such, I would also propose that the idea of protecting yourself from catching the yearly flu through an outside-in medical intervention be wholly unfounded if seasonal sloughing is the mechanism through which these symptoms are experienced and not by the invasion of a new microorganism or virus.

Instead, I believe these seasonal changes or the environmental signals that affect the trees and rabbits are also affecting humans.

Our bodies react to the sun being a further distance away from our place on earth. Our bodies react to the diminishing internal production of vitamin D. Our bodies react to lower levels of energy and moisture in the air through the form of dissipating heat and humidity. Our bodies react to our circadian rhythm changing based on fewer hours of sunlight. Our bodies react to the changes in temperature and barometric pressure. These, along with the more subtle changes that our bodies respond to from season to season, trigger changes within us that have been programmed after millions of years to initiate a cascade of symptoms to purge our internal biomes, much like the cascade launched as trees begin to change and drop their leaves or disperse seeds.

It is already well-known and understood that the human body uses environmental signals to adapt to things like hormone production. Based on specific factors, like the presence of light for example, in the case of our bodies' melatonin production (the hormone that makes you sleepy and controls your circadian rhythm), these hormones can be directly influenced. We know that the production of melatonin can also be negatively affected by blue light in particular, which is why the light from an electronic device at nighttime can be so disruptive to our sleep quality. Light inhibits the natural production of melatonin, so melatonin production is designed to pick up in the evening when the sun starts to set and exposure to light is reduced. This increased melatonin production helps our bodies fall into natural sleep — it's how our circadian rhythm is programmed. Melatonin is also partially converted into DMT while we sleep, which is an essential component of our ability to dream.

So, the understanding that our body reacts to environmental signals with hormonal and cellular changes is not something new or completely abstract; however, it *is new* to suggest that our bodies *react to these seasonal differences by purposely recalibrating our internal bacterial environments to suit them better.*

Stated again, it is my opinion that our bodies respond and react to subtle seasonal changes, such as changes in atmospheric energy and the presence and distance of electromagnetic impulses from the sun, prompting our bodies to create different internal environments to adapt to each season most efficiently. This process requires the expulsion of excess old and unbeneficial biotic organisms in the form of bacteria and weak or dead linings of internal tissue; a process carried out by triggering a cascade of internal cleaning processes that happen simultaneously to both expel the portion of our biome not suited to the new environment and initiate an internal spring cleaning of old tissue and waste products of cellular cycling. So, this Seasonal Sloughing is of our old tissues, as well as the internal biome that is no longer suited to the new environment.

When we express symptoms of a seasonal cold or flu, if seasonal sloughing is true, then these symptoms are not due to opportunistic entities infiltrating our bodies with new subtle mutations; rather, they are the body's natural process of seasonal sloughing and cleaning to properly adapt our internal environments to new external environments. I am not saying that there is *never* a bacterial or viral transmission of an illness through the traditional means of opportunistic infection, but I believe it is erroneous that this is the mechanism responsible for incidences of natural immune adaptation in regard to the formation of the idea of the symptoms of a seasonal cold or flu.

OPPORTUNISTIC INFECTION

On that topic, I would like to address opportunistic infections and opportunistic illnesses because I do believe these to be true mechanisms of illness in some instances; however, in the general scheme of how we understand illness and sickness, I believe we have attached far too many expressions of symptoms to these elusive foreign entities.

I believe that the traditional idea of infections by a pathogen entering the system are reserved for more novel and deadly situations when we are presented with a novel pathogen that does not exist in nature, such as anthrax or lab-created illnesses, or in hospitals when someone is contaminated with a superbug during medical treatment. In these instances, the mechanism of illness and death is more likely due to the toxin portion of that novel substance or bacteria or by it being presented to a portion of the body that bypasses the immune system, such as an open wound during surgery, or by the sheer amount of something entering a system that cannot be processed efficiently, such as consuming E. coli. But in a normal environmental aspect of daily living, I do not believe that the opportunistic cold and flu cascade is a true explanation for most of what we have long considered to be cold and flu symptoms.

To further our understanding of this, let's consider the current understanding of gut health.

THE GUT BIOME

Our gut health has a huge impact on our overall health and is dictated by the composition of our gut biome. This has been well-known in the nutritional world for many years, but it's only been in the last few decades that the health-gut connection has become a mainstream idea.

The bacterial composition inside of our gut (gut biome) is responsible for maintaining a balance that is essential for appropriate gut health and nutrient absorption. These bacterial entities break down food and release chemicals that have a direct impact on our nutrient uptake, as well as our global and mental health. When our gut biome is thrown off by using antibiotics or eating toxic, processed, and chemical-filled foods, there's a change in the internal gut environment due to these toxins, which results in a change in our gut efficiency and function. This change in our internal environment causes a change in the balance of microorganisms inside the gut and changes the balance of bacteria. This altered balance is responsible for many different health conditions like Crohn's, IBS, diverticulitis, and leaky gut, and contributes to almost every digestive tract pathology we know of. However, new research is now showing that it also has an impact on things seemingly far removed, like our mental health. These new implications come in the wake of the fairly recent discovery that we actually have *neurons* (brain cells) inside our gut that form a direct line of communication between the two that has now been called the *gut-brain connection.*

It turns out that the bacteria inside our gut are not only important for appropriate digestion and proper nutritional absorption but also for our mental health, so much so that we've started looking at feeding the gut with beneficial bacteria and replenishing the gut biome to treat mental health conditions! Ten years ago, suggesting feeding properly balanced bacteria to our gut to treat mood disorders would have gotten you laughed out of any medical school classroom, but now it's groundbreaking.

By looking at this single example of one area of our internal biome, we can see that the proper balance of our internal biomes has an immense effect on our health in multiple ways we are only just recently beginning to understand — and this is with only one region of our internal biomes being studied — we have countless more that haven't even been considered!

Though our understanding of the gut biome is still very much in its infancy, why would we assume that the rest of our bodies' systems don't have their own equally important internal biomes? It is more likely than not that the principle of an internal organ-specific bacterial biomes is universal, and we just haven't thought to look anywhere else yet except the gut.

When we observe the rest of the organs and systems in the human body, it is well understood that every internal and external surface of our body is completely lined with bacteria and microorganisms of some sort. From the skin inside of our nose to the epithelial cells inside of our mouths, to the tissue in our trachea, all the way down inside our lungs, and to the internal tube that makes up our excretory tract. Every single organ we have, to some varying degree, is lined with microorganisms that are designed to aid in the health and balance of that organ, contributing to the global health of the system, and function of our body as a whole. Humans and bacteria have formed a symbiotic relationship with each other, and the function and survival of the human species are dependent on this relationship to the same extent that humans are dependent on oxygen and water. Like it or not, despite how much current politics wants you to bathe in hand sanitizer, these microorganisms have developed over millennia to form a mutually beneficial relationship with us. And strangely, *we need them more than they need us.*

We provide them a solid, comfortable, and warm environment in which to live and reproduce, while the products of their reproduction and their presence on and in our bodies function to aid our bodies' own processes in fundamental ways and protect us from the harshness of the external environment.

It is the currently accepted understanding in microbiology that one of the organelles inside of every one of our human cells, called the mitochondria, (functions as the powerhouse of the cell and is responsible for creating the energy each cell is dependent on to function and perform the basic tasks of life called ATP), is expected to have once been an independent entity or bacteria of some sort that, through the process of phagocytosis (cellular eating,) was absorbed into the cell and somehow, instead of being broken down and consumed, began to lend the cell its functional abilities. These borrowed functions became so fundamental within the cell that this newly consumed bacteria integrated into the human cell permanently and became a part of the cell's genetic coding, ultimately integrating into the blueprint of every cell. From this mysterious time forward, during every cellular division, a mitochondrion would replicate and be present in each new cell. This outside entity became an inseparable part of the cell because of its benefits to the cell function. A symbiotic relationship formed between the two entities that was so strong they merged into a single entity, which is now the base structure of every tissue in our bodies.

At the very base of the human cell, we already see that part of our *human cells* exists as a cell of a *different entity*, presumably a bacterium of some sort, that has been so important that it has become a consistently replicated portion of ourselves for the entirety of human existence. — Good thing we didn't have hand sanitizer millions of years ago!

Now, if we can understand the necessity of a mutually beneficial relationship with various bacteria on a gut biome level and a fundamental cellular level and agree that outside bacterial entities are interdependent and hugely related to our own cellular and global function, then it's not a far stretch to accept the idea that our bodies would respond to subtle signals of environmental changes, such as seasonal changes, to work with the external and internal bacterial entities to adapt our internal biomes to best suit our external environments. It would make sense that there would be an evolutionary mechanism in place to allow us to customize our biomes to suit the specific environment we are in — especially when living in a region that has drastic differences from season to season, so that we, as humans, can so readily explore new terrains and adapt more effectively to new and novel climates. It would also make sense that to customize these biomes, we must shed the old biome that is no longer suited somehow.

In some areas of the world, seasons have vast differences from one to the next, such as here in Canada. These seasonal differences result in drastic differences in vitamin D availability, differences in atmospheric moisture, and differences in atmospheric heat, in which our body must find a way to regulate heat in different ways, such as gaining higher levels of subcutaneous body fat for insulation. On top of that, our bodies have to change internal processes to aid in regulating and responding to changes in moisture, changes in free and available electric energy in the air, and changes in hours of sunlight, which alters the intensity of the energy being given off by the sun, changes in food availability and types of food we have access to and nutrient sources, etc.

Though this may seem extensive, it is, in reality, just a short general list of the most noticeable differences in seasons. However, it is likely that the extent of environmental signals our bodies are innately tuned to respond to go much deeper and are much more robust than what we are currently aware of and likely expand into categories that we currently can't even imagine. As a species, humans have survived and evolved to the extent we have because of our unique ability to adapt to such varying climates and circumstances. Still, our interdependence and interaction with environmental signals is what makes us a *part of nature*, not some strange entity that exists outside of it.

Despite being intrinsically connected to nature and all organisms sharing some ability to adapt, it has been said that humans still stand alone as the most adaptive species on the planet. Humans can live in highly varying climates — not only as native cultures that grew up in those climates — but also as visitors or immigrants who may have been born and raised in a vastly different climate and region of the world. If an individual was born in Africa, they can come to Canada and still survive and thrive in this environment despite some short-term discomfort and adaptation. The same concept applies to a Canadian who moves to Africa. This level of adaptability would not be possible if we did not have regulatory mechanisms built inside our immune systems and cellular structures that allow us to alter our internal environments to effectively adapt us to new external environments.

The internal regulation system of seasonal sloughing also allows us to integrate a new environment's newly adapted bacterial biome into our own in the most beneficial and seamless way. Though sometimes, depending on how different the new bacterial biome may be, this process can be uncomfortable for a short time, we nevertheless can still achieve this adaptation for all except the most extreme cases.

When we are introduced to a new water system — for example, if an American were to travel to Mexico or Iran for the first time — that individual may become sick when first exposed to the bacteria, spores, and microorganisms in the water. However, if these individuals remain in this new area, they will eventually be able to drink the water safely and not get sick, just like the people who have lived there their whole lives. This is the process of integration and adapting the internal biome to fit the environment best — and the portion of this theory that I am calling Continuous Bacterial Priming — which is carried out by the same mechanism as the seasonal sloughing mechanisms, only to different environmental signals that are not based on seasonal changes.

Seasonal changes present environmental signals that communicate to our body that a change is required in our internal systems. This transition can be a seamless one, or it can be quite jarring, depending on the individual's overall state of health and the extent to which their unique internal biome has to shift to accommodate the required adaptation.

You may have noticed some individuals get seasonal colds and cases of flu multiple times a year while others seem never to get them at all, or one person gets sick on vacation from the food while another who ate the same food does not. At first glance, this would look like a problem for my theory and would seem, on the surface, to lend credence to the invasion aspect of germ theory. However, it also makes complete sense within the Seasonal Sloughing and Continuous Bacterial Priming Theories.

The reason for this difference in experience from one person to the next is that each person's unique internal cellular health plays a huge role in helping us either go through this transition smoothly or violently. Put quite simply, the healthier and more properly balanced a system is, or the closer it is to what is required, the less it needs to change to adapt, and the more efficiently it can do so without an uncomfortable and dramatic event.

Suppose you are an individual who leads a very healthy lifestyle. You consume proper healthy, whole foods, and have a proper chemical and electrical balance inside of your body. You consistently force your body to adapt to change through exercise and novel experiences. In that case, your body will need to do less to accommodate the upcoming seasons — it will need to shed and expel less damaged and discarded bacterial residue in preparation. An overall healthy lifestyle will result in an overall healthy body, and minimal transitions will be needed because you will be consistently pruning off your old, weak tissues and cells through the concept discussed in the next chapter so that these sloughing procedures will be carried out by the cells with little effort and high efficiency. On the other side of the spectrum, if your body is in an unhealthy and unregulated state, already struggling to adapt to the functions of life and the current environment, and not receiving constant controlled stress to prune off old tissues, then the transition and process of sloughing off and reconstructing your internal environment for the upcoming season may present as a more aggressive transitional period with a higher expression of symptoms. The overall lack of health and efficiency in the body systems will be exaggerated during this time, and higher levels of tissue waste and bacterial debris will need to be discharged, resulting in a fever, cough, runny nose, and phlegm — aka cold and flu symptoms.

If your body is healthy and with low amounts of toxic cellular damage and leftover debris, the sloughing process will be easy and with minor symptoms, if any, since your body contains the necessary building blocks for proper cellular functions and does not have an overabundance of old debris. However, if your body is going through a more violent transition, it is likely due to low internal cellular health due to nutritional deficiencies, toxic exposure, low levels of daily internal cellular recycling through exercise, or exposure to a completely new and novel environment with a noticeably new biome to adapt to, such as traveling to a new climate.

If the latter is the case, then your body has to do more to integrate, regulate, and adapt to the new environment because it does not have the appropriate cellular memory of previous regulations to that same climate or may be in the process of integrating completely new environmental microorganisms and biomes as a whole. This is why when people move to new areas, they can experience new allergies or even new illnesses for a short period while their bodies excrete the old, no longer suitable biome and create a new one as their bodies and the new environment assimilate into each other. These new illnesses are often short-lived and resolve after the body fully integrates and adapts to the new environment and climate.

CURRENT COMPETING THEORIES

The views I have presented above differ drastically from the mainstream-held ideas about colds, cases of flu, and germ invasion theory in a few fundamental ways. Let's look at the two competing theories of human immunity that are recognized in our existing literature.

The more dominant of these two theories was created by a scientist named Pasteur and is held onto by the mainstream with a death grip due to its usefulness to the pharmaceutical companies in an effort to force their products onto you in a never-ending parade of outside-in cures. This useful theory is called the Germ Theory. The other, older, more scientifically valid but less accepted theory inspired by the work of scientist Antione Bechamp is called Terrain Theory. Let's take a look at both and see where, if possible, the Seasonal Sloughing and Continuous Bacterial Priming theories can fill the gaps.

GERM THEORY

Germ theory, the current model heavily endorsed by the opinions and private interests of our time, dictates that the human immune system is a weak and vulnerable defense mechanism that is highly susceptible to invasion by external forces at all times. These external forces include all bacteria and viruses that we "catch" from other people or from any variety of objects we come in contact with in our external environment. Once we are exposed to these opportunistic and pathological entities, our weak immune system fights to defeat them but is typically overpowered, and we become ill unless we have come in contact with this exact version of the pathogen previously and have a memory of it in our immune system archives. The illness we experience is our bodies' desperate attempts to expel and fight the invaders who made it past our first defenses. In this model, we are in a constant battle with the natural world.

According to germ theory, when we are exposed to or "catch" a virus or bacterial infection, it invades our body. It begins to reproduce rapidly while our body fights desperately to categorize and destroy it. This is a process that happens daily and often results in symptomatic expressions such as fever, running nose, coughing, etc., as we veer closer to losing the battle, only to be miraculously delivered from this looming catastrophe, usually with help of some medicine given to us by our doctors aka the priests of the Religion of Medicine.

Though I believe this theory to be incomplete, at least up until recently, it was thought that our body could fight these invaders with a fairly high success rate and that, as humans, we actually had a very robust and powerful immune system that was built through constant and *necessary* exposure to environmental bacteria, viruses, and pathogens of all kinds.

It *was* believed that playing in the dirt, getting dirty, and exposing our children to these pathogens helped prime them to have healthy immune systems as adults, and it was looked at as not only favorable but *mandatory*. It was also believed that we received our original protection through the antibodies passed on from our mothers' breast milk, which is why it was so important to breastfeed when possible, to supply children with the tools necessary to be healthy in the environment they were to grow up in.

Though the science of all the above beliefs is still very true, and nothing has disproved any of the above about immune system development, many powerful industries and political movements have slowly, and now almost completely, changed the story and used germ theory to form a modern weapon against our psychology and health. The true tenets embedded in Germ Theory that allowed us to trust our immune system and live a healthy, natural life in accordance with nature — despite us believing we were being constantly attacked — have been all but completely abolished since this mysterious virus hit in 2019. The process of stripping humans of faith in their natural immune system has been happening slowly and consciously for decades, as you will see, it has reached its apex in our current political time, leaving the majority of the unsuspecting public in constant and utter terror of the natural world.

In this slow and purposeful split from nature over the last few decades, before it reached its apex in previous years, there has been huge lobbying from various industries ¾ such as the baby formula companies which led to public manipulation using things like articles in pediatric magazines claiming breastfeeding should no longer be thought of or referred to as natural, and that formula was considered a *better* option than breast milk. They somehow were able to trick the world into believing chemical baby formula is healthier and more properly balanced for our babies than the innate intelligence that exists within breast milk. This idea is being pushed to the public when in fact, breast milk is so intelligent that the mother's nipple has tiny receptors within it that register the chemical content of the baby's saliva to inform the mother's body about which nutrients and minerals the baby is lacking, prompting the mother's breast milk to automatically recalibrate to provide a milk rich in those specific things.

If you somehow have been tricked into thinking that a prepackaged, dried, generic baby protein shake is better for your children, it's not your fault. It's because you have been systematically brainwashed. I am not here to shame anyone about this topic. If you are an individual who struggled to produce milk and needed to use formula for that or any other reason, then that is completely ok, and you should be proud of everything you did to make sure your baby was fed and loved. What I am saying, though, is that the idea that formula is interchangeable with breast milk is erroneous and we have been led to believe it for reasons much less wholesome than pediatric health.

This is just one example of a simple way Germ Theory has been used as a weapon to slowly unravel and destroy our understanding of natural health and natural immunity in seemingly unrelated areas— the slow and subtle deconstruction of the idea that we have natural,

God-given functions in our bodies that are proficient and competent and that we have a robust and adaptive immune system has been slowly phasing out over decades. This slow but continuous conditioning has led people to panic when their body shows a symptom and sprint to stop it, take yearly flu shots, dose up on cold medicine, avoid their loved ones, and reduce their own oxygen intake using toxic and bacteria-covered masks, all in the name of health.

In the last four years, this theory has been taken to its epoch, transforming into the current rhetoric of the mainstream media and top doctors that our body can no longer fight any novel virus or bacteria whatsoever nor fight the same fights we have been winning against opportunistic invaders since the dawn of time. The story is that we are all in incredible amounts of danger unless we cover our faces and sign up for a punch pass card that provides gene therapy to force our bodies to create and produce the very thing we are supposed to be running scared from. This insult to our natural bodily function is the ignorance towards breast milk all over again, only on steroids.

Our immune system, according to the weaponized version of germ theory, is a fumbling, blundering, helpless system that needs our external assistance to function properly. This external assistance has been coming in the form of magic pills and potions for decades and now has transformed into magic injections. Corporations are now altering our immune function and gene expression *permanently* with every dose given in an attempt to supposedly help our fumbling immune system to do what it has done at an extremely high level of efficiency for millions of years.

Viruses come and go, but gene therapies are permanent.

This level of irrational rationalization has only been made possible through the systematic weaponization of Germ Theory over many years and the subsequent conditioning of our minds and belief systems to accept its end conclusions.

While in its original version, Germ theory may have been an honest and balanced theory, it has now become an overly convenient theory used in a capitalist-based medical model to fuel its products by proposing that all danger comes from the outside ¾ therefore, all help must also come from the outside.

If your medical model is designed to funnel money to huge companies that make products that can be patented, then you have to convince the public that it is only through these patented products that our helpless bodies can become and remain healthy.

Without germ theory, modern medicine would not be able to function in the way that it does. Modern pharmaceutical companies would not be able to have a death grip on the human population because the human population would no longer need them for the majority of the illnesses that we see today. In fact, if it weren't for Germ Theory, most of the illnesses we see today *wouldn't even exist.*

In contrast to germ theory, there is one other competing model of illness that we will take a look at that has been gaining attention in the natural health communities over the last decade but has lost almost all support from the various medical industries. This theory, despite a very low acceptance rate in modern mainstream medicine, has a large amount of scientific data to support it now, just as it did 100 years ago when the scientist Pasteur potentially plagiarized the work of this theory's leading scientist and stole the spotlight to create

Germ Theory and win the support of the medical machine. This competing theory is called Terrain Theory.

TERRAIN THEORY

Terrain Theory starts with a single question: if two people live in the same house and eat at the same table, consume the same food, breathe the same air, and do the same job, why does one get sick in a certain situation and the other doesn't? The answer, according to Terrain Theory, is that our *internal environments are the primary dictating factors for opportunistic infections and illness*. In short, our own internal and cellular health is responsible for us either being the sick one in the household or the not sick one.

Sounds familiar?

Terrain Theory believes that our internal health is the most important factor that predicts and regulates our ability to adapt to pressures and foreign entities in an external environment. It is this underlying truth that is used as the backbone of my proposed Seasonal Sloughing Theory and what I believe to be the foundation of overall immune function. In essence, I believe Terrain Theory provides the primary truth about immune system function, and I believe the Seasonal Sloughing and Continuous Bacterial Priming theories to be adjunct theories that fill in gaps of Terrain Theory that had not been previously discussed or understood, while Germ theory, in its original form, provides the mechanism of immune system diversification.

Now, the above may be a slightly simplified explanation of Terrain Theory, but it is easy to see that it is quite logical. We know enough about human health at this point that we are very aware that individual health is a massive predictor of mortality and illness rates among a population. This places the greatest predictor of illness into the hands and habits of the ones that are ill in all the ways that I previously stated were factors in predicting whether an individual was to experience a fairly aggressive or a fairly mild transition to seasonal changes and new environments. The indicators and base levels of health predictors are shared between the theories, which is why they work so well in conjunction with each other.

Again, as stated, the Terrain Theory is true, but in my opinion, it is incomplete. But at the same time, in some instances, Germ Theory is also true but incomplete — as mentioned previously. If you eat a big ol' burger containing E. coli bacteria, you will likely become sick. This fact fits both Germ Theory and Seasonal Sloughing Theory. The extent to which you get sick and your body's ability to fight off infection would fall into Terrain Theory and Seasonal Sloughing Theory. Because Germ Theory can be true in situations of high-density bacterial ingestion, it doesn't mean that it applies to all other aspects of the immune system, especially not seasonal changes. Germ Theory is a necessary understanding for some instances, but the weaponized and hyperbolized version of it presented today is an over-exaggeration of its application and an over-generalization of its effects.

Terrain Theory as a whole, then, applies to a much more logical and robust area of our immune function and, in my opinion, is a more accurate description of how our immune systems function. (If you eat

McDonalds every day and sit on the couch, it's pretty obvious your immune system will not function at its highest capacity.) So, despite these two theories both being true and relevant in certain situations, I believe that between the two of them, there was still a missing piece of that puzzle that could serve to join them in a more accurate and universal understanding of human immune function. I believe that the missing pieces are the Seasonal Sloughing/ Continuous Bacterial Priming Theories.

Terrain Theory demonstrates the individual differences from person to person and the importance of overall individual health as a predictor of immune function. Germ Theory accounts for how we can get sick when exposed to high levels of pathogens through diet or environmental exposure and how our immune system broadens when introduced to new pathogens; however, neither of these theories accurately explains what is happening regarding seasonal colds and cases of flu and our body's symptomatic expression while adapting to new environmental signals. Only Seasonal Sloughing and Continuous Bacterial Priming can explain how and why we constantly and predictably undergo sloughing behavior and re-prime our internal environments based on the new external environmental signals we are exposed to.

Humans are designed to adapt and change with the seasons and new environments as a natural process, just like every other living creature on earth.

Seasonal Sloughing Theory is designed to fill the gap between the two currently existing models and tie them together into a global immune system understanding. I believe that every year, the bacteria, viruses, and various other life forms that make up the environmental biome evolve, mutate, and change. Our bodies constantly interact with these new variations of organisms, along with the cyclical and seasonal changes and environmental stimuli, interpreting and responding to them to upgrade our internal environment to better suit the external environment at all times. I believe that with seasonal changes in temperature, sun ray intensity, humidity, free electromagnetic energy, pollen, spores, etc., our bodies undergo natural updates to our systems. These updates include the sloughing of the previous internal biome that is no longer compatible with the new external biome and integrating the new mutations and environmental organisms into our new internal biomes. Through this process, our bodies internally shed our skin like a snake and re-calibrate in a way that allows for optimal function in the new environment and with the new microorganisms present. This process happens continually year-round when exposed to any new environmental organisms but is most aggressive and noticeable during seasonal changes because this is the time when the largest environmental cues trigger the calculated transition and are directly affected by our cellular health and habits. This explains why we have phrases in our culture like, "Don't go outside without a jacket or you will catch a cold," or why your grandma always used to warn you that if you go outside with wet hair, you will catch pneumonia. When we are exposed to cold weather, it is an environmental trigger that informs our body that it is time to recalibrate for the cold. Even the name of this process is called catching a *cold*. This demonstrates that the phenomenon has intuitively been understood in its connection but not in its sequela.

So, when you go outside in the cold and you catch a cold, you are not getting sick; rather, your body has been triggered by external stimuli to undergo the shedding process of your old internal environment and restructuring it to better protect you in the new environment. The symptoms of a cold are the symptoms of your body strategically burning off, coughing out, and expelling the old bacterial and micro-organism biome to make room for the new one. The symptoms are proof of your body's intelligence and ability to adapt, not a sign of your body's weakness and failure to protect you.

(*Side note: This may also be the reason that purposeful cold and heat exposure, in the form of cold plunges and saunas, may have such a favorable effect on the immune system.)

The seasonal flu follows the same process, except it is your body integrating the new mutated forms of the environmental microorganisms into your new biome, along with the signals and stimuli from the environment itself. Every single year, we have a new flu that is marketed as a dangerous new pathogen out to kill us. However, what is happening is the microorganisms that exist in the environment are continuing to evolve and adapt, just as we are. Our body, when it comes into contact with them, is taking them in and upgrading our biome *using* the new microorganisms as building blocks to allow us to coexist better while fine-tuning that biome to best protect us from the different variables present in our current climates. The symptoms of the seasonal flu, just like the seasonal cold, are the natural expulsion mechanism that our body innately possesses to expel the old biome efficiently, as well as mitigate how much of the new novel versions of these microorganisms are in our system while our body integrates them into its biome. Once the integration is complete, symptoms reduce and stop altogether, and we now have an upgraded internal biome to coexist with the upgraded external biome harmoniously.

This process also happens every single time we go to a new environment, such a foreign country. When we first arrive, especially if it is vastly different in its external biome from where our biome is used to being, then it is likely that when we eat the food and drink the water, we will get sick, aka we will be exposed to new microorganisms that our body must integrate. Sometimes, if the biome is so different that our bodies cannot adapt quickly enough, it can lead to severe illness or death; however, in most cases, even if the symptoms are aggressive, our bodies will adapt to the new biome and integrate the new microorganism and environmental markers into our own over a short time. Regardless of the severity, the process of the illness is the same. Our bodies are working to integrate the new microorganisms into our internal biome to allow us to exist and function optimally in the new environment while expelling through multiple pathways all excess and no longer needed materials. This is Continuous Bacterial Priming.

The intelligence built into our bodies and existing within our innate immune systems allows us to adapt and evolve with the microorganisms around us constantly and within the climate around us. For hundreds of years, scientists have marveled over how human beings can adapt to so many environments and still thrive. I believe the Seasonal Sloughing/Continuous Bacterial Priming Theories hold the keys to this mystery.

I also sincerely hope that Seasonal Sloughing Theory holds the key to the disassembling of the Germ Theory as a weapon and the power it has over us all as a result. Once we understand how powerful we are, how innately intelligent and competent our bodies are, and that every process in our body has a purpose, we can begin to work with helping the body and honoring it instead of trying to work against it and override it.

FURTHER IMPLICATIONS AND CONSIDERATIONS OF THIS THEORY:

COMMUNITY & PROPER IMMUNE FUNCTION

Once we understand the implications of Seasonal Sloughing Theory and Continuous Bacterial Priming Theory, such as the body's innate ability to integrate the microorganisms of the external environment into our internal environments to build a robust and healthy internal biome and immune system, we must look at other ways in which this process may aid in the formation of both our individual, as well as our collective health.

When we live in isolation, we are exposed only to the microorganisms within our own body and immediate environment. If we have a dog or a cat, then we get exposure to their biome as well, which helps our biome to have a small amount of diversity to work with. However, once our bodies adapt to our limited environment, they work to optimize our internal biome within this environment, allowing us to adapt in a way that helps us thrive in our bubble and our bubble only. We become isolated to a small number of microorganisms and environmental variation, and we slowly become hyper-specialized to survive in this limited environment.

But what happens when we finally leave our bubble?

Limiting our exposure to diverse environmental microorganisms allows us to adapt to a limited environmental biome. If we restrict this exposure for an extended period, it results in a significantly less diverse internal microorganism biome. When we have a less diverse internal biome, it results in a less robust internal protection system and less variation in external environments that we can be exposed to without experiencing symptoms.

To help understand this better, pretend we are out in the streets of New York and think of every unique microorganism inside of our biome as a member of a different gang. If we have a member of a certain gang inside of us, and we run into that gang in the outside world, then this internal member we have in our tribe can act as the ambassador and safely harbor our passage through their designated block without much harm or hassle. If we have a robust internal tribe, and we have a unique ambassador for every one of the gangs that exist in New York, then we can walk safely down pretty much any street at any time and not have to worry. Even if we happen to come across someone who is from a novel or new gang in town, once they realize our affiliation with all the other pre-existing gangs in town, they will not attempt to cause us any harm. Even if they do, they will be quickly put in their place.

So, a robust and diverse internal biome results in our ability to safely handle almost all external environments and microorganisms that we come in contact with and allows us to quickly and efficiently handle new microorganisms when they are presented because of our immunological diversity and robust previous affiliations. But what happens if we try to walk down the streets of Brooklyn at night with no protection, no connections — not even the slightest bit of familiarity with them because we haven't left our safe little bubble in far too long?

Well, we would probably be more like Steve Erkel walking down an alley alone in the dark.

When we remain in isolation from the germs of others in the outside world, we cultivate an internal biome that has the protective capacity of a wet paper bag. Put very plainly, if you limit your exposure to external germs for an extended period, your body will not be adequately adapted to the outside environment and the updated environmental biome. It will become hyper-specialized to your controlled environment, and any exposure that strays from that will create a massive shock to your system and you will "get sick."

This means that every time you are exposed to a new microorganism or a new mutation of an old microorganism, your body will have to struggle much more aggressively to integrate the new microorganism into your biome, which will result in you experiencing much more aggressive symptoms than you normally would, and likely, more often than you normally would. This will result in a much more severe expression of symptoms to even mild and normally inert external pathogens than it would for a person who had maintained consistent exposure to new, novel pathogens.

Essentially, leaving your house and walking through a crowd of people in your hometown will have the equivalent effect on your immune system as flying to India for the first time and walking through the crowded market. Your internal biome will have lost its robustness and diversity, meaning you will have to undergo intense and uncomfortable upgrades through exposure to get it back, and these will present to you as intense illnesses.

The good news is our bodies are extremely adaptive. Despite the loss of robust protection, you will eventually be able to adapt and return to normal health if you maintain exposure and allow yourself to power through the discomfort. Think of this in a similar way to what happens to a person's gut biome after a round of antibiotics and how you need to reseed the gut with healthy probiotics to avoid further health complications. If, however, you get scared of the symptoms of your "illnesses" and retreat into isolation, the problem will only be compounded the longer you stay in your bubble. Eventually, you will begin to see other people and the natural world as dangerous and aggressively point your finger at them as the problem. After all, as long as you don't leave your bubble, you don't get sick ... So it must be *other people that are the problem and making you sick, right?* Wrong.

This is the inherent necessity of community and the inherent risk of isolation. Further, this is also the inherent risk of the larger idea of believing that exposure to microorganisms through people or nature is a bad thing. (Get out that hand sanitizer, amiright?!) The more people we are around on a consistent basis, the more variations of microorganisms and diverse biomes we are exposed to, and the more novel environments we can experience, then the more robust and diverse our protection will become. These result in huge upgrades to our immune systems and internal biomes constantly, which outlines the fundamental process of forming robust, resilient, and healthy immune systems and maintaining a balance as part of your environment.

We have always known that in almost all areas of life, diversity is key. If you want a healthy, robust financial portfolio, you need diversity of investments and income streams; if you want a healthy body, you need diversity of movement and nutrient intake; if you want a well-balanced education, you need diversity of information and class material; if you want to be a great musician, you need diversity of musical training and genre study; if you want a robust immune system and a well-calibrated internal biome, you need diversity of exposure.

Period.

DIFFERENT FOODS FOR DIFFERENT SEASONS

This portion of the chapter is not linked with the concrete theories listed above; rather, it is an intellectual continuation regarding another possible way our bodies may be designed to work in unity with seasonal cycles. I have no real data or discovered evidence to support the following musings. However, logically and intuitively, I believe that there is likely more truth to it than I am even considering.

Think of the following as an Einstein-style thought experiment.

Consider This

I believe the foods we are designed to eat in the wintertime, based on the limited availability of crops and cultivated preserving methods (before worldwide shipment of goods year-round), are more mucus-forming and heartier by design, to aid in our formation of internal mucous membranes, which may serve a purpose in protecting us from the harsh winter climates and allow enhanced internal thermal conservation.

The types of foods that would have been more readily available to us in winter climates historically, such as stews, soups, bread, and meats, along with canned and pickled goods and root vegetables, not only are considered to be mucus-forming but also have the added benefit of having increased caloric densities. This high caloric density, when consumed, carries with it a heightened glycemic load and higher insulin production, which would allow for greater nutrients in smaller portions but would encourage more sloth-like and conservative physical behavior upon consumption. This would have the natural result of lowering our productivity levels and making active working hours match, potentially in a strategic way, the reduced daylight hours, and free electric energy available in the air during the cold winter months.

In the same way that I demonstrated that seasonal sloughing creates a similarity between human seasonal changes and those of trees or rabbits, I believe the changes in food during the winter months form a similarity between humans and bears.

Though bears eat high amounts of calories in the months leading up to winter and then have a full hibernation season, I believe humans have an approximate version of that in that we eat higher-density foods in winter and have pseudo-hibernation qualities daily during winter months. Another comparison for ease of understanding is the relationship between fasting and intermittent fasting. The first is the full expression of fasting for a prolonged period, representing the bear, and the second is a daily mini fasting that takes qualities of the true form but in a smaller, more habitual way, representing the human.

I believe this to be the effect of the higher caloric, mucus-forming foods we traditionally consume in winter. They allow us to integrate mini-hibernation qualities into our lifestyles during the cold and dark months to conserve energy and keep us in tune with seasonal rhythms.

Consuming high amounts of mucus-forming food long term and throughout all seasons may result in some potentially long-term negative effects on our health; however, if done in the winter months and cycled out in the summer months, it may have positive, protective benefits.

As mentioned above, mucus-forming and high-caloric foods may create enhanced levels of insulation from the environment internally (through mucous membranes) and externally (in the form of subcutaneous fat under the skin). The types of foods that would have traditionally been available to us during the cold winter months would be typically high-fat, high-carbohydrate, high-protein, calorie-dense foods. Access to fresh fruits and vegetables would have been impossible during these times.

The negative effect of these foods we see in our current society is due to overconsumption and over-availability year-round. We have more food availability now than at any other time in our history. Despite this, if consumed in the proper seasons, these high-caloric, mucus-forming foods may actually have an evolutionary and dietary benefit. The physiological effects of these foods may be designed to increase cholesterol and increase coronary atherosclerosis short term purposely to create short-term insulation to our entire system to help protect us from the extreme cold and dryness of the winter season, as well as priming us to operate at a lower environmental energy reserve. Again, I would like to say that this is a contemplative topic. I have no proof of these claims; I am only bringing to the surface ideas that I believe have solid logic and require further investigation.

When exposed to dry environments, we often experience cracking in various places of our dermal tissue or skin cells. Our lips, mouths, hands, faces, and all other areas of our skin exposed to the cold air's extreme dryness tend to break down and become susceptible to cracking and damage. It's possible that mucus-forming foods are designed to line our internal organs with an appropriate layer of mucus to protect against the harsh exposure to dry, cold wintertime environments. This may be why there is a somewhat instantaneous effect when we eat mucus-forming foods, and it may be tied to our ability to survive such harsh climates. This could also play into the proposed cycles of things like blood pressure and cholesterol levels, depending on the time of year in which they are measured.

Have you ever noticed that many people, especially elderly people, get very sick and pass away right around Christmas? This, in general, could be a very open-ended conversation as the factors that are involved in this phenomenon are staggering; however, I believe that part of the reason we see this phenomenon is that medications affect our bodies very differently depending on the season in which we are taking them and the season in which we were diagnosed with whatever condition they are designed to treat.

Now, that may seem like a mouthful, but bear with me.

I propose that changes in an individual's blood pressure and heart rate in the summer versus the winter months would lead to specific incidences in which, during a particular month, an individual may present with higher blood pressure than normal, based on their response to seasonal cycles and environmental changes. (Everyone knows that if you have a heart problem, taking too hot of a bath can be dangerous due to increased heart rate and blood pressure.) During that time, the doctor measuring the blood pressure may find it appropriate to prescribe blood pressure-lowering medication. This may be appropriate and necessary for that individual at that specific moment; however, if their blood pressure was high during the summer time as a response to environmental cues, and then winter comes around, the blood pressure naturally lowers itself as a response (as a hypothetical but possible example), then as a natural lowering process takes place, the added medication the individual is on may lose its positive benefit and combine with the natural decrease, could result in that patients' blood pressure dropping to a dangerous level and may put that patient at risk.

These phenomena and the interaction of these cycles with medication may be a large contributor to the fact that something called *Iatrogenic death*, which is death by medical error, is the *third leading cause of death in North America*. Again, the examples above are hypothetical but logically sound and, to this point in medical literature, uninvestigated or even considered.

Another recorded phenomenon in which this idea can be demonstrated is the phenomenon that the majority of drug overdoses happen in an area that is unfamiliar to the user. Studies have shown that individuals can have a significantly higher dose of a drug when they are in a familiar environment with lower subjective and physiological effects than when they are in an unfamiliar environment. This suggests that area recognition can help a person handle and process the external toxin more efficiently.

So, if alterations of toxin uptake and regulation can occur based on familiarity with the environment and can be so extreme that they can affect an individual's ability to process and metabolize drugs in their system, then things like seasonal changes could very well present a significantly higher alteration to the average person's bodily systems than we think or have ever investigated.

Considering this, we would also be behooved to consider that if a patient goes to a new clinic to see a specialist or doctor for the first time, there could presumably be a difference in their regulatory diagnostic readouts based on the unfamiliar territory. Their blood pressure may be off the charts because of the stress of the new environment, not because they were low on Beta-blockers.

These factors are not considered in any scientific analysis within the medical communities; however, further investigation and controlled studies of these subtle but possibly significant factors need to be done to understand the human body and health fully, along with its relationship to the world around us.

We are not an island, so we shouldn't be treated like one. We are an integral and active participant in nature, and thus, nature is an integral and active participant in us.

CHAPTER 19

BASE LEVEL OF INJURY / GUIDED INFLAMMATION

As with the Seasonal Sloughing and Continuous Bacterial Priming theories, this next theory that I am about to present is, to the best of my knowledge, another original idea based on insight gained by studying and working with the human body on multiple levels over the years.

The Base Level of Injury Theory, or Guided Inflammation Theory, is based on the idea that to maintain appropriate levels of cellular turnover and appropriate cellular health and function in our bodies, there needs to be a base level of injury or destructive stimuli presented in consistent, controlled, and varied ways to reach to all areas of our bodies to maintain consistent cellular turnover and limit old, mutated, or sub-optimal cells from causing stress, dysfunction, and disease. This controlled turnover is needed to maintain and continue the process of appropriate cellular destruction and regeneration, using controlled stress as a catalyst for turning older, weaker cells into new, vibrant ones. In short, we require an appropriate amount of stress and cellular destruction through minor, function-based injury to prune off old and weak cells and stimulate the growth of new, fresh, healthy cells.

This theory can be demonstrated through multiple avenues because it is a universal principle consistent throughout bodies and demonstrated throughout our lifetimes. Think about how many times a child falls or is minimally injured in a given week. Now think about how many times your Uncle Joe is in his 40s…. Now think about how many times Grandma Betty is in her 80s. As we age, we not only reduce our exposure to physically stressful situations, but we also limit our controlled internal pruning by limiting ALL forms of physical stress ¾ and I'm sure we have all heard the saying, if you don't use it, you lose it; but how about we change that idea to if we don't consistently work something, it will get old, stale, and dysfunctional. Think about the car you have parked in your garage that hasn't been running in years every mechanic will tell you that is much worse for the car than driving it every day, even if the driving it puts it at risk of normal wear and tear.

An example in the human body that is very easy to follow is the process that takes place during exercise. When we exercise a muscle — whether that muscle is the quadriceps, biceps, or heart — the exercises that prove to be the most effective at cultivating overall health are ones that are controlled, consistent, and progressive in intensity over time. Consistent exercise provides enough stimuli to elicit enough muscle exertion and controlled stress that it pushes a person slightly past their normal level of comfort or average ability at that time. Regardless of your motivation or intentions, you can't get results at the gym by going one time and doing an extremely intense level of exercise that is vastly outside of what your body can handle. It simply isn't a recipe for success.

Instead of positive results, it will inevitably lead to injury and high levels of tissue destruction, which will take significantly longer to recover from and potentially cause serious, long-term problems. In comparison, positive and progressive results come from calculated, moderated effort over an extended period, consistently providing a small, destructive stimulus and giving the body ample time to recover before delivering the next controlled stimulus.

Positive, progressive results in a biological system require low-level stress followed by time and nutrients to recover.

If you go to the gym consistently and appropriately and push your muscles through a properly constructed building phase in which you slowly work up the number of reps and the amount of sets you do each time you go to the gym while allowing appropriate rest days in between and feeding your body the proper nutrients needed for your muscles to grow and recover, then you will start to see appropriate gains, and positive, measurable progress.

Once your body gets primed and accustomed to doing this type of exercise, your muscles will start to respond, and you will soon notice that you can handle a higher capacity of stress and intensity without the same risk of injury that you faced when first starting. As an experienced lifter, you can start to push those muscles harder and harder while lowering the risk of injury due to positive adaptation, allowing you to reap the benefits of those muscles constantly being stressed and systematically pushed past their limit just slightly, resulting in building those muscles stronger and turning those muscles over. Constant stress on the muscle causes constant muscle cell turnover. There isn't enough time without being worked for old, stagnant muscle cells to exist unchecked. These are the principles of exercise physiology but also the principles of baseline human physiology.

All physiological systems respond to stress. Whether that stress is positive or negative depends on a) how much stress is applied, b) how long it is applied, c) how close that stress is to what your body can handle easily already, and d) if your body has the appropriate internal building blocks to recover after it has faced the stress. Our bodies are designed to adapt and overcome stress, as long as that stress isn't too far outside of what we are already used to. This is the fundamental importance of the Base Level of Injury theory, in that the more controlled and purposeful stress we encounter, not only do we gain higher levels of adaptive abilities, but we also maintain a healthier level of strong, functional cells while forcing the weaker ones to be pruned off due to their inability to deal with the consistent, controlled stress loads.

When you exercise any muscle, including your heart, the stress of the exercise damages the tissues to a small degree, sending inflammatory cells to the area. The damage to the tissue affects the old and weak tissue in the area first, which allows the inflammatory cells to clean up the debris and initiate the growth and formation of new cells to take the place of the old and now dead cells while healing the healthy tissues that are still strong enough to be used.

This process systematically guides inflammation to different areas of the body to force those areas to be triaged and pruned, turning over the cells before they can become stagnant and dysfunctional. When used strategically and purposefully, the Base Level of Injury theory mechanisms can become a conscious health practice by deliberately guiding the inflammation to all systems and areas of our body through varied exposures to stress. This allows us to utilize their pruning capabilities , take control of our cellular health, and aid the body in maintaining proper cell turnover throughout our lives.

We can direct inflammation through systematic, minor injuries from varied stimuli to affect varied areas of our physiology, which will proactively recycle old cells in each one of these areas and replace them with new, healthy ones each day.

Using exercise as the theme because it's one of the main ways we can actively apply the Guided Inflammation Theory, let's look at how these same mechanisms affect cardiovascular health through exercise.

Have you ever noticed that whenever you go for your first couple runs of the season, or you have your hardest cardiovascular workout in a while and push yourself a bit harder than normal, your throat tastes metallic? Almost like you can taste very slight amounts of blood?

What has happened is the increased expansion pressure on the trachea and the increased force of air moving through the throat and into the lungs creates a higher abrasive force than your body is used to. These abrasive and expansion forces of air being forced in and out of your lungs and blood flushing into the cells lining the organs and tissues involved in this process cause a base level of injury to those cells.

Despite this being damaging in nature, this abrasive force actually acts as a positive stimulus to the area by breaking down some of the tissue in that area and stimulating it to be replaced by younger, stronger cellular tissue. It is the destructive forces of abrasion and expansion that stimulate the body into a constructive response. Basically, the internal signal we receive is that we are facing a much more stressful environment, so to be better suited to face it in the future we better get stronger.

Buck up, champ.

When we break down small portions of the body in a natural way, and a way they're designed to be broken down(through challenging them with an activity they are designed to do), the guided and natural destruction of those cells results in a positive turnover and the construction of new, stronger tissues in that area. I believe that this Base Level of Injury is required for maintaining appropriate cellular health throughout the entire body and through all the bodily systems. If we consciously and purposefully harness it, we can use guided inflammation to create an effective and predictable healthcare paradigm and wellness philosophy.

I believe this extends even further past exercise. I consider this idea to be universal and to also exist in the forms of small, non-problematic and non-complicated injuries like scraping our knees or bumping our legs into bikes and tree branches. When you are active, you *always* have a number of scrapes and bruises, meaning you always tend to have some small injury somewhere. This, counterintuitively, I believe, is helpful in cultivating long-term physiological health.

If you look at athletic individuals (and all individuals who maintain moderate to high levels of physical exercise), they are always dealing with some small level of discomfort or injury. I believe that these small, inconsequential injuries are part of the body's process of consistently and constantly turning over tissue and are, therefore, fundamental in preventing stagnation of tissue and disease development. I would also like to note that I am using the term injury here in a slightly different way than we are used to. I am not referring to high-level injuries or things that would pull an athlete out of the game for weeks of recovery. Instead, I am speaking of the fact that all injuries are of the same nature: tissue damage from stress. Only the injury I am referring to is a very small level of damage so as not to change or hinder overall function.

So, let's say for another example, if you have a balanced, healthy habit of doing breathwork, cardiovascular exercise, and anaerobic exercise — whether that be yoga, weightlifting, or a combination of the two, or any consistent sport — these activities allow your body to move consistently under stress, and result in a systematic and continuous guiding of inflammation to all the different areas and systems of your body that are involved in processing that particular stress. This is like creating a comprehensive cleansing habit for your body by using your inflammatory cells to sweep their way through your bodily systems on a consistent basis, resulting in the breakdown of old, less healthy cells throughout your body and replacing them with new, young, vibrant, healthy cells. If you create a comprehensive cleansing program that routinely causes a base level of injury to all of the major systems of your body, then you can create a consistent physiological form of cleaning house.

Without this Base Level of Injury/Guided Inflammation, our cells effectively begin to exist for too long in certain areas, which opens them to becoming weak and prone to mutation and dysfunction. These alterations in old cells could result in the replication of dysfunctional cells and eventually lead to disease. It is my belief that areas that are not constantly turning over due to a Base Level of Injury or undergoing the process of Guided Inflammation on a somewhat regular basis become the cellular equivalent of what you would find in a still lake or lagoon. Without appropriate cellular turnover, these stagnant bodies of water, or cells, become the bodies where disease and infectious agents grow.

So not only is this an effective health strategy, but it's also a necessity if we want to protect against tissue decay and mutation in the body. Our bodies require a constant Base Level of Injury among all our tissues and systems to prune off weak and old cells before they become diseased and to replace them with new, healthy tissues. Without a Base Level of Injury, our tissues and cells have no controlled stimulation or stress that pushes the cellular turnover process in a proactive and consistent way.

This lack of stress allows old cells to exist without challenge and continue to replicate longer than they should in a healthy, active body. This leads to a greater chance of disease and mutations of cells being replicated from these old cells. The Base Level of Injury and Guided Inflammation processes are fundamental in maintaining and regulating the health and function of every single organ, muscle, and system of the body and can be systematically directed in a controlled way to manage and maintain human cellular health and function. This is one of the underlying reasons that consistent exercise, facing novel stimuli, performing daily work, and consistent performing of skills and functions throughout our lives is so important, and has such a big impact on predicting positive health outcomes. Inflammation is an incredibly important and necessary process in our bodies — we have to learn how to guide it through maintaining a consistent and varied Base Level of Injury, but also know how to shut it off so that we have enough time to recover.

LET'S TALK INFLAMMATION:

We have been led astray.
Again.

As with all things in the body, inflammation is somewhat misunderstood. We hear about inflammation in current health and mainstream sources, and it's a bit of a buzzword — often linked to negative conditions or chronic disease states; however, that is only really the case when we are speaking of *chronic inflammation*. Outside of chronic and uncontrolled inflammation, the process of inflammation itself is fundamentally one of the most important processes in the body.

Inflammation is caused by the migration of certain inflammatory agents to the area called neutrophils, eosinophils, lymphocytes, plasma cells, and histiocytes. Each one of these cells has a different job and different functions that are integral to the immune system, as well as to the inflammatory response in our bodies. These particular cells are also part of the body's overall surveillance system. Their job is to migrate to the area that has undergone some form of stress or injury and triage the situation. If a foreign entity or invader is causing the inflammation, such as an antigen spoken about in the last chapter (foreign bacteria or virus), then these cells send signals to the B cells and T cells to ready the body's military, and begin bringing in troops to fight.

When we develop an immunity to something, it is because these cells have met a similar invader in our bodies before and have stored an extensive report on them; we have specific fighters that were created just for that particular invader (these were the members of our robust posse that kept us safe in the streets of Brooklyn talked about in the previous chapter), so it's the inflammatory cells that quarterback the process of investigating the cause of stress in our bodies, and calling in the necessary troops to fight.

If the inflammation is caused by an injury instead, then these inflammatory cells again triage, but this time, they send signals to work with the platelets in the blood to create a barrier to stop blood loss and any further fluid loss. If the inflammation is from a toxin, then these cells send signals to wall off the toxins and begin metabolizing the toxins as soon as possible. Basically, without inflammation, we do not have a functioning immune system or protective system from any injury or toxic exposure.

Inflammation is the bodies healing mechanisms in action, and it is actually our best friend, not our enemy ¾ the only thing that makes it an enemy is our society's lack of understanding of it and insistence on consuming toxins that cause inflammation every single day.

This information is all common knowledge and true in all medical textbooks; however, what the Base Level of Injury theory suggests is that a small amount of *appropriate* injury is needed to keep our cells turning over at a healthy rate and to prevent pooling and stagnation, which leads to disease and mutations such as cancer. As long as the injuries are small and constantly cycling, then this is a healthy process for our body, very similar to pruning a plant or conducting controlled burns in areas that are at risk of forest fires. This controlled damage recycles and prunes away old cells and stimulates the growth of new ones. This process, over time, creates an efficient system that is constantly being tested and pushed towards efficiency while not allowing old or dysfunctional cells to multiply, and decreasing stagnation of cellular waste products.

The cleanest water is always in an area where the stream is constantly moving. Without controlled injury causing guided and cycling inflammation, cellular waste products pool in certain areas, and the body has the potential to allow toxins to pool and harmful cellular mutations to happen. These toxins multiply, and these old cells begin to mutate. The last thing we would want is for those cells, exposed to so many toxins and harboring mutations, to be allowed to multiply unchecked ¾ with guided inflammation, we can constantly send out triage teams to all these different areas to clean houses.

This is the way inflammation is *supposed* to work in our bodies.

Inflammatory cells are one of our main lines of defense and a fundamental part of our internal surveillance system. Problems arise when we stay in states of chronic inflammation. Chronic inflammation, which, like all other forms of chronic stress, leads to overstimulation of these inflammatory signals, causing a consistently overactive response, ultimately leading to a hyperactive immune system (auto-immune disorders, food intolerance allergies, etc.) and an overstimulated sympathetic nervous system (diffuse pain conditions such as fibromyalgia, high blood pressure, anxiety, etc.). These two states, over time, lead to destructive physical processes and become conditions such as inflammatory forms of arthritis, Crohn's, diverticulitis, coronary artery disease, and potentially even cancer. Controlled burns that lose control and become forest fires.

What we know about chronic inflammation is that it is the *effect* of some other cause. The cause is the problem; the effect is not.

Attempting to treat chronic inflammation with pharmaceutical chemicals that synthetically block inflammation in the body and decrease inflammatory markers is like attempting to fight a war by firing all the sergeants in your military. It not only completely misses the cause (as with almost all allopathic forms of treatment), but it also decreases your body's ability to properly heal and triage dangerous events in the body. Most relevant to the last few years, *taking anti-inflammatory medication lowers your immune system and slows your healing.*

Instead, using the Base Level of Injury Theory as a platform and the Guided Inflammation theory as a blueprint, we could work to properly direct inflammation to different areas of the body by stimulating those areas in a natural way to trigger the process of pruning old cells and cycling stagnant fluids, thus using the body's natural processes to recycle and cleanse the cells in the affected area, and throughout the whole body.

The fundamental idea of this theory has been something we have intuitively understood for a long time, but to the best of my knowledge, it has never been written down on paper like this. We know that if you want better lung capacity and health, you do cardiovascular exercise. But what we didn't realize is that cardiovascular exercise helps to prune off and destroy unhealthy lung cells while stimulating and growing new healthy ones in their place. Understanding that this is a universal principle for all areas and systems of the body provides us with a path to follow to begin to restore our health and flush out areas of stagnation within ourselves. It gives us a concrete health reason to exercise, instead of our goals always being about fat loss or aesthetics.

This theory also provides another reason why consistent chiropractic adjustments can help create overall greater health in an individual: Each area adjusted is moved in a way that it does not usually move on a daily basis. This movement causes stimulation to the area and a small amount of inflammation as those inflammatory cells then migrate to that area and triage. This is where the *directed* portion of directed inflammation comes from. Along with exercise, chiropractic provides us with another tool that allows us to guide the body and tell it where to direct inflammation so that the body can triage the specified area and trigger the processes to calibrate and heal it. Using a chiropractic adjustment, we can quite literally guide someone's internal surveillance system to check in on all important areas of their body regularly. Consistent check-in and triaging of the whole body will increase the efficiency and appropriate recycling of cells throughout the entire body, which, if done consistently, just like exercise, will lead to a higher level of global, systemic cellular health.

Much like how they are using prolotherapy now to stimulate inflammation inside a joint, we are using our hands to do the same thing in a much less invasive way. This is one of the reasons that chiropractic medicine is such an effective form of healthcare for injury rehabilitation and the *cultivation and maintenance of overall health.*

Using the Base Level of Injury theory as a backbone and applying it through the Guided Inflammation theory while understanding the appropriate and natural cycles our bodies go through in response to seasons, stress, and internal and external environmental stimuli through the Seasonal Sloughing and Continuous Bacterial Priming theories, along with the information presented in the first section of this book, we now have a guide to follow to consciously and purposefully cultivate our health. This information puts the power of your health and wellness back into your hands in a way that we have not had in the entirety of my lifetime, nor that of my parents or grandparents.

Understanding the basic principles of proper bodily function and how those functions are expressed and guided allows us to become our own health gurus. We no longer need to rely on "experts" and top doctors to tell us how our bodies work. Even more importantly, you now hold in your hands an instruction manual to begin to guide your immune system to create a healthier and more robust you.

You now, more than ever, have the tools to better understand your own body and begin to reclaim your own health.

I hope you feel empowered. Because you should.

PART III

WHAT NOW?

CHAPTER 20

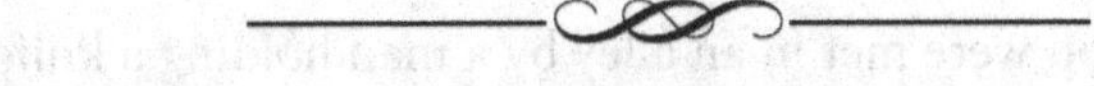

IT'S TIME TO REWRITE OUR STORY

I'm sure you have heard the phrase, "We are a collection of the stories we tell ourselves," But have you ever stopped and considered the *true* significance of that before now? The truth is the stories we tell ourselves not only make up what we consider to be our identities but also the entirety of what we consider to be true in the world. Our stories form the backbone of our realities, and what we know forms what we think is possible.

Our self-image is just an idea we uphold, as is our perspective of every person, place, thing, or event we ever encounter or experience. These ideas are usually a synthesis of multiple events that have occurred in our lives, how we feel about them, what we have been told about them, and how we believe others would or do feel about them. We know ourselves almost entirely in relation or comparison to other people, and we see the world in relation or comparison to our learned ideals and subjective memories of previous events, whether real or fictional.

When we look back on events in our lives, we first judge them, then we judge ourselves, weighing our actions in relation to how we currently think or feel we should have acted or how we envision another person would have reacted instead.

Say, for example, at one point, you were mugged. Walking home from the bar, you were met in an alley by a man holding a knife and asking for your wallet and watch. You gave it to him. Frightened, you did what you were told and froze. Though not what you may have wished you would have done, your actions may have just saved your life.

Regardless of whether your actions were right or wrong, what happens afterward? Often, the emotions quickly change from the instant sensation of relief to something that feels much worse ¾ like shame.

But why would this happen? After all, you just avoided physical harm and got away safely. Well because you likely are weighing your actions against what you *believe* someone else would have done. You find a way to idealize an alternate response, and your shame forces you to dwell on it.

Maybe it's because Arnold Schwarzenegger is your hero.

Maybe you are a big Connor McGregor fan.

Maybe you have spent years with posters on your walls of Bruce Lee or Clint Eastwood. Maybe you were even the high school tough guy or girl.

Looking back on the incident, you begin to draw comparisons. You feel shame in the contrast between how you think one of these idealized people would have responded and how you feel you did. This results in a feeling of weakness and increasingly negative self-image. Ideas begin to float in your mind, convincing yourself that you are a coward, too weak or scared to stand up for yourself when it matters. After years of this self-deprecating story, you notice that you have slowly become the image you perceived of yourself. You have avoided all conflict out of fear and a woefully low self-esteem. You have become the coward you once thought you were by repeating the story of how weak and helpless you are in times of crisis.

Now, walking home years later, from the corner of your eye, you spot an elderly woman as a man walks up, pushes her to the ground, and grabs her purse. Next thing you know... *BOOM!* Without even thinking, the man is on the ground, and you have the old lady in your arms as you pick her up and begin yelling for help. As the would-be mugger sees the attention you are drawing, he flees. Shaking and confused, you try to hide your pulsing heartbeat from the lady as you gather every bit of strength you have to be a calm voice for her, as she is clearly much more shaken up than even you. She thanks you sincerely, and you walk her to her bus stop and part ways.

By the time you get home, you are replaying the incident in your mind, thinking, "How the heck did I do that? I'm just a coward; I don't even know what happened."

So... what did happen?

Because you didn't have enough time to think, there was no time to review the story you have been telling yourself. You reacted out of a gut impulse to help someone you knew needed it.

The most un-cowardly thing possible.

Even though you didn't know it, it was something you would have always done but had never faced a situation that forced you. Helping someone who needs it is a lot different than getting into a knife fight with an armed man over a wallet and watch.

Using an objective lens to view this made-up story, we can see that in both situations, the individual probably *did the right thing*; however, because the first incident doesn't fit with what we see in action movies about idealized characters, the individual created a negative self-image based around their inability to live up to the fictional construction of bravery. They created a story based on cherry-picked ideals to create a situation and a memory that elicited a negative emotional response and became a catalyst for the construction of a negative self-image over time.

This story became a prison and created a disempowered self-image that had a far-reaching negative impact for years. Not realizing that the response to being mugged was actually the right one, this story of shame and weakness became a broken record playing on a loop, distracting from the truth. But how do you think this fictional version of you would feel about yourself after the second incident?

It's likely you would feel brave, perhaps confused, but vindicated. Seeing that you acted in a way that was noble and brave, perhaps you begin to enjoy the feeling of this safety. Your confidence climbs. Your chin feels a bit stronger. You may even sign up for self-defense classes and start walking with your head a little higher. Your posture changes, and you start making more eye contact with everyone you pass.

You have changed your entire life simply because you have changed your story.

One incident can write your entire story if you let it, and one decision can re-write it. The power is always in your own hands and your mind.

This situation shows the malleability of events in our memory, and how our feelings towards those events form the basis of our past, and shape how we perceive the present.

We all have key events that tend to repeat in our heads.

Some good.

Some may not be so good.

And some are downright terrible.

Have you noticed which ones play most often? Yup. The terrible ones.

As humans, our survival instincts pre-program us to fixate on the bad. This is a big problem for mental health in and of itself; however, another problem is the way in which we tend to change and exaggerate events. We either wrongfully remember events in the past or dramatically catastrophize events we think will happen in the future. We use these events on repeat in our heads to fuel bitterness, anger, and our unique, varied experiences of depression.

These events become reminders as validation for the negative feelings we carry with us. They create self-fulfilling prophecies. Not only about our self-image, but also about our health. But what would happen if we decided to change the stories? Is it possible to rewrite the past and, therefore, rewrite our present experience of it and our future expression of it?

Yes. It absolutely is.

When you begin to look at the events of your life not as a helpless victim but as an active agent, you can play detective and begin looking for clues for something you may have missed or colored in a way that may not have been truly accurate, such as our faulty ideas about how our bodies function.

Suppose you keep replaying an event or idea over and over in your mind, always exaggerating the same conclusion. In that case, you may miss the hidden opportunity that event or idea presents. You also may be completely missing the big picture, just as a detective may miss finding the real culprit if they've already decided who the guilty party is before even starting the investigation.

If we have repeated the same stories about ourselves and our bodies our whole lives, assuming that what we think we know and what we have been told is true, *we may just be missing some of the most important and empowering knowledge about who and what we actually are.* If we always look in one direction, we miss everything in the other.

We have been trained to believe a certain version of ourselves as humans. We have been taught through school, movies, media, and cultural norms that we are a weak and helpless species. We have been convinced that our bodies decay rapidly, and there isn't anything we can do about it. We have been taught to fear relentless and elusive entities that, at any moment, can invade our bodies and cause unpredictable and irreversible damage. We have been told the story that we desperately need help from people much smarter than us to eventually use the miracle of science to cure all the big, bad boogiemen of the body that, unless they do, will inevitably kill us and everyone we know.

Worst of all, we have been convinced that there is nothing about the human body and human health that hasn't already been discovered and studied, and that anything worth our attention would be told to us by the priests of the Religion of Science.

But I ask again, what would happen if we changed that story?

Just like the second version of you presented above that saved the helpless grandma, over time, I believe with enough wisdom and intention; we can lose the negative self-image instilled by these stories and rewrite a new one of empowerment beyond what we can even imagine. We don't have to live as the scared, weak, and cowardly version of ourselves that serves the interests of the world's pharmaceutical giants; instead, we can realize that just like we always could, we can heal ourselves from much more than we think we can. We can also begin to see how much magic exists in this world and within our bodies and develop a more profound understanding of what it means to be human.

THE UNIQUENESS OF YOU

To add an extra layer to this, if you look at every human on earth, it isn't hard to see that every single one of us has had, and will have, a dramatically different experience of life. Our experience, when compared to anyone else, will never be replicated or even approximated by another human being ever again. There are endless events, experiences, and emotions that happen throughout our lifetime, and it is, quite literally, mathematically impossible for somebody to have the same arrangement of events, emotions, and experiences that you have experienced in your life. This fact alone demonstrates how no amount of cookie-cutter information on health and wellness could ever serve every one of us in the same way because each one of us is so distinctly unique.

Along with being unique in life experiences, we are also unique sparks of divine energy, having a completely novel and unrepeatable influence on the world we are living in through our everyday interactions. Using this wisdom, I believe it is easy to see that each one of us fits the categories of both being created and being a creator. As such, each one of us really does have a divine purpose here.

When we look at the particle makeup of each one of us, we are made up of trillions upon trillions of particles that are all being recycled and replaced every single second of the day with particles from outside of ourselves. We discussed a macro version of this in the cycling of bacteria in the Seasonal Sloughing and Continuous Bacterial Priming theory, as well the recycling and replacing of old damaged cells with new healthy ones in the Base Level of Injury theory — but there's more to it than that on a more microscopic level.

Every second of every day, we are taking in new particles and atoms from the atmosphere around us in exchange for expelling particles and atoms that previously existed within us back to the outside world.

These particles we take in don't just appear from the ether. Instead, these particles came from somewhere or something else before us. They were previously arranged in a different pattern, as a different force of matter, and likely in a different state of matter, inside another person, place, or thing.

We may have carbon atoms or nitrogen atoms inside of us currently that once existed inside of a wolf, or were once part of a tree, or a snail, or even existed as a droplet that showered the streets in the beautiful rainfall last night.

We have such a vast array of particles inside of us that assemble and disassemble in ever-changing patterns from the moment of our conception to the decay of the last tiny fragment of our bodies long after we are forgotten about. Given how mathematically impossible it would be for somebody to have the same arrangement and order of life experiences as somebody else, it would be even more unthinkable for *any other human being to be made up of the exact particle makeup that you are at this moment, or ever have been or will be in your life.* You aren't even the same you that you were yesterday!

Inside of you, you have stars, you have animals, you have plants, you have oceans. You then ARE all these things to some degree or another, and you are ever changing.

I suggest you take a moment to really fathom the enormity of this.

Within you, you have all that exists ¾ and within all that exists, there is part of you. Part of your essence is in every corner of existence, and the essence of every corner of existence is right inside of you.

To put this into perspective, let's look at just a simple deck of cards. A deck of playing cards only has 52 individual cards ¾ much less than the total number of your life experiences and unthinkably less than the total number of individual particles in your body by multiple orders of magnitude; however, working out the math of shuffling that deck of only 52 cards, which represents 52 unique life experiences or 52 unique particles in your body, we use the mathematical calculation of the factorial of 52! The factorial of 52! calculates how many unique variations and unique arrangements of those 52 cards would be possible. Now prepare yourself, because when you do this calculation the results are, quite frankly, much harder to comprehend than I could ever have imagined.

If a new shuffle were done of these 52 cards every single second since the big bang (13.8 billion years ago), *then by now, only less than 0.1 percent of all possible shuffle arrangements would have been completed*! This means that every single time you shuffle a deck of cards, even if you did it one million times per second for the rest of your life, you would likely *never* get the same order twice!

....

.........WHAT?!

THAT'S ONLY 52 CARDS! Our body contains trillions of cells that have been recycled from countless places and are consistently being rearranged every millisecond. Furthermore, 52 unique experiences in someone's life can happen before they have even finished their coffee in the morning each and every single day!

This is mind-blowing. So next time someone tells you that you aren't special or acts like the same advice should be taken and followed by every person in the world, hand them a deck of cards and tell them to go kick rocks!

Every single one of us is a unique particle makeup, living a unique experience with unfathomable power and the ability to create our own realities. The stories we have been taught to tell ourselves are of false histories and limiting beliefs. We have been drilled since we were children to internalize the idea of fitting in and adopting self-deprecating limits. We have been told magic doesn't exist, we cannot change the world, and we are *only human.*

It's time to re-write that story. Both for ourselves as unique and powerful individuals and for humanity as a whole.

We are not *only* human; we are *incredibly human.*

CHAPTER 21

IN HIS IMAGE

Don't we know we are like God? And like God, we have the ability to create at will, perhaps more than we have ever imagined.

This was the true message of Jesus, and what all esoteric wisdom is based upon. In John 14:12 Jesus states "Truly, truly I say to you, whoever believes in me will also do the works that I do, and greater works than these will he do, because I am going to the Father." Jesus told us outright that through our belief and understanding, we could be capable of even more than he was.

Look around.

Look at what we are capable of and what each one of us has been able to do within our own unique lives. Even the humblest of persons can see the miracles that they have been a part of and the unexplainable events they have witnessed. These events can be big, like a premonition in a dream that comes true the following day, or small, like the text of someone coming through moments after you thought of them. Our lives do not fit within the bleak and narrow parameters that modern science tries to force us into.

Look at every other living species on this earth and compare them with yourself. Every living creature is a miracle in and of itself, and every one of them deserves appreciation for their unique and magnificent qualities, but no other animal on earth comes close to the wonderful and diverse abilities of humans.

We are a *reflection of God*, created in his image. We have been told this from the beginning, but have we not realized the significance? It seems we haven't. Created in his image does not just mean we physically look like God ¾ instead it means that within us, our entire make-up is a reflection and projection of God. As above, so below. The perfect ideal projected down to the physical world. God is our original blueprint, and we are made in his image. If we could grasp this, then we would understand that we are capable of anything we can imagine.

Instead, we have all forgotten the unique abilities to create that we have been gifted to us all, and in doing so, we have thrown away the inherent power we each have that comes with those gifts ¾ It would also seem that there is a concerted effort from a small group of wealthy people to stop us from ever remembering this and learning who we are and what we are capable of.

The weak, sick, and divided need a constant source of reassurance and constant intervention from outside sources to quell their anxieties and heal their infirmities . The empowered, however, do not.

What the empowered have is wisdom about themselves and about the natural processes that take place on our planet and in our bodies, as well as how those processes shape and affect our lives. The empowered have an understanding that no one and no thing exists as an island, but instead, all things exist in relation and conjunction with everything else. The laws of this world are based on cause and effect. When these relationships are unknown, the effects may seem unpredictable and scary; however, when these relationships are understood, the effects are predictable, and the causes can be managed to sway the desired outcome in the direction you choose. Arthur C. Clarke said that magic is just science we have not understood yet. I will take this a step further and say that science is just a natural law that has been repackaged and used for profit. Now that we can see it for what it is, we can unpackage it and use the gifts we were all given.

So, what more do we need to prove to ourselves that we are more than we once believed?

We can already do almost anything we desire and turn almost any thought into reality. We have hundreds of millions of self-help books about our ability to attract and create what we want in this world, so much so that it has become a saturated and overprinted market. It's become common knowledge, almost to a cliche degree, that we are literal magnets and can attract and create the life we want based on our thoughts, intentions, and actions. As a species, we can already do *almost anything*. The only thing limiting us is the purposeful withholding of information that can and will allow us to expand our abilities and self-understanding even more. The following steps in our evolution require free access to information. ALL information, not just the approved article and algorithms on our social media and search engine platforms, and that information includes who and what we really are.

We go through life like everything is boring and limited. Yet, we hear stories of supposedly impossible feats, like a desperate mother picking up a car to save their newborn baby or people with psychic and extrasensory abilities like remote viewing, and we pass them off as too weird to believe. Meanwhile, our primal and innate memory of these dormant abilities within ourselves has caused our society to become obsessed with superhero movies and stories about magic. We watch these movies and read these stories obsessively, forgetting that all those things have been real for countless people throughout history. These myths and legends come from somewhere deeply connected to the history of the human race. We can imagine them so tangibly, but we can't believe they could be talking about *us*. This is the power of controlling the narrative for hundreds of years. Every generation gets further from the truth, and eventually, old events fall into legend.

Now, after so many generations and such expansive levels of brainwashing that we have faced, the biggest hurdle we have in transforming our lives is *our own beliefs*. We have been raised on propaganda that continues to inundate us with stories and warnings about how fragile we are. From every corner of our realities, we have continuous messages of our inadequacies. These clever sources of media and fable work tirelessly to remind us that *we are only humans*. Our creative will is stifled by our exploited reactions to fear. We fear change, we fear illness, we fear death, we fear war, we fear our neighbors, we fear losing our jobs, we fear the food we eat, we fear germs, we fear everything we interact with daily, and when we grow so tired of it that we think about standing up and making a change, we fear failure, and we fear ridicule.

We have been coaxed into a life in which we are given false options of comfort and convinced that it is the epitome of success and happiness to be an obedient and agreeable good boy or girl. We live in a world where we are bombarded with so much fear and uncertainty of the future that we are too scared to make any moves, even if they lead us to a better one. Change is now the enemy because it could disrupt the comfort of the safe routine in which we are living. But what we don't understand is that simple changes, even in our mindsets, can be a catalyst to the complete rewriting of our destinies.

Comfort may be comfortable, but it may also be a form of submission to a life and a future that, whether you are an active agent in it or not, is destined to change and disrupt your routine, one way or another. I don't know about you, but I would rather try to write my destiny based on the stories I choose than have someone else write it for me. Especially when those currently writing it seem to be trying to actively write us all *out* of the story completely.

Secondary to this fear of change is our lack of belief. Our lack of belief ranges from simply not believing in the power we hold within ourselves to make simple changes in our lives, such as in our careers or relationships, to the more insidious implications that have massive effects on our confidence and self-worth, such as the lack of belief that the power that made the body can heal the body; or that we are *only human*. Our lack of belief in ourselves is founded upon our *lack of understanding of who and what we truly are.* And that is the crux of the situation, and where I hope this book will help.

If we can finally understand that we are individual emanations of God, made in his image and with his abilities to create and that we are not only participants in this world but *creators* of it, then our limiting beliefs would dissolve and would be replaced with a newfound sense of confidence and purpose. Once we understand that we are more powerful than we had previously imagined, our ability to face challenges without the fear of failure and discomfort will become a natural and obvious default. From there, we can stand on a whole new foundation of self-knowledge and self-confidence that would free us from the bonds of a life filled with anxiety.

Along with this new foundation, we can safeguard this confidence by understanding that the only reason our belief in ourselves was ever attacked is that it was the only way to control us. They needed to lower our will and lower our confidence in ourselves, because we are too powerful if they don't.

Depressed confidence and self-belief lead to depressed people.

Depressed people are easy to manipulate into believing they are worthless little accidents and inherently flawed.

Empowered beings are not.

If we can begin to understand that we do not need laser vision or the ability to fly to be like God and that simply existing the way we do is already profoundly God-like, then we can begin to cultivate and expand our power. Our lives may seem common, but that is only because all the magic has been systematically and strategically stripped out of our minds, so we no longer see it in front of us. But if you start to look for it, you will realize it's there.

It's always been there.

If we take a moment to change our lens when we look around and within us, we will see the truth that has been there all along ¾ we are gods, and we are magic. Whether in tiny or profound ways, we use magic to create every single day, and we exist as profound mirrors of the divine.

Everything that has been created by humans, from the vehicles we drive to the phones we talk on to the buildings that tower over our downtowns and create beautiful city skylines ¾ they have all been created by the collective *us*.

God created all, and from there, in his image, we have continued to create as well. We humans have co-created the reality we experience, and we co-create our own bodies and health every day. Humans as a species have collectively created these things, and we as individuals create the lens through which we experience and interpret these things and events every single day, including the vehicle in which we use to experience them. We were blessed with this body and these unique abilities, and to not use them would be a waste of the most precious gifts imaginable.

We are divine beings, and we are active agents in this world. It's time we open to our potential and start acting the part.

This is, after all, a call to action.

AFTERWORD FROM THE AUTHOR

This book is an accumulation of the things I've learned, discovered, seen, read, and experienced in my life up until this moment in my story. Though, as stated previously it is not an exhaustive catalog, I hope it served its purpose in piquing your interests and speaking to the mind, body, and soul of you, the reader. This book is a guide and explanation of human health and the human experience as I see it, touching on all aspects: mental, physical, emotional, energetic, and spiritual. It has taken me years to get this out and available to the public — not just years of writing and intention to concretely lay out my thoughts and beliefs for others, but also years of editing and waiting for the right time to share it with the ones I love, and the world.

This book is the culmination of many years of passionate and extensive study of all the areas of the human condition and human health that I have been lucky enough to have access to. It is intended to serve as a guide and provide a new lens for every individual who reads it to view themselves, their bodies, and their place in the natural world in a new and more powerful way. I hope this lens positively changes and colors how you see the enigma of human health, consciousness, and experience. Most of all, I hope it provides you with the tools you need to regain control over your health and start your journey of radical self-empowerment.

I believe in my heart that this book provides unique and important missing pieces of information that have never been available to the public about the intricacies of human health. I hope these missing pieces help us all increase our collective understanding of the human body so we can move further toward a state of true and natural health, both within ourselves and on this planet as a whole. I hope that we can understand how we, as the spectators of this world, are also active participants in this play unfolding around and within us.

I hope that these words find you well and that who you are after reading this book is a more empowered and excited version of yourself as you take this information and walk with it as a guide to facing the ups and downs of this life with confidence in yourself, and your body, and that it may contribute in some way to your experience on this earth being one of genuine love, excitement, appreciation, health, gratitude, and divinely created joy.

May you live in harmony and peace with this beautiful world, and may we work together to tend to its gardens as we each fall in love with the process of tending to our own. Thank you for reading.

Now, go create a life that inspires you.

Yours truly,
Dr. Nicholas James Nelson.